Color Atlas and Text of

DENTAL
AND MAXILLO-FACIAL
IMPLANTOLOGY

John A. Hobkirk
PhD, BDS, FDSRCS (Eng & Ed)
Professor of Prosthetic Dentistry
Eastman Dental Institute
for Oral Health Care Sciences
University of London

Roger M. Watson
MDS, BDS, FDSRCS (Eng)
Professor of Prosthetic Dentistry
King's College School of Medicine &
Dentistry
University of London

Tomas Albrektsson
MD, PhD (*Author of Principles of Osseointegration Section*)
Professor & Chairman
Department of Handicap Research
University of Göteborg
Sweden

Contributor:

Geoffrey H. Forman
BDS, MBBS, FDSRCS (Eng)
Consultant Oral & Maxillo-Facial Surgeon
King's College School of Medicine &
Dentistry
King's College Hospital

Foreword by:

George A. Zarb
BCHD, DDS, MS, FRCD, Dr.Odont.
Professor & Head of Prosthodontics,
University of Toronto
Canada

M Mosby-Wolfe

London Baltimore Bogotá Boston Buenos Aires Caracas Carlsbad, CA Chicago Madrid Mexico City Milan Naples, FL New York Philadelphia St. Louis Sydney Tokyo Toronto Wiesbaden

Project Manager:	Anton Lawrencepulle
Developmental Editor	Claire Hooper
Cover Design:	Pete Wilder
Illustration:	Lynda Payne
Production:	Michael Heath
Index:	Jill Halliday
Publisher:	Geoff Greenwood

Published in 1995 by Mosby-Wolfe, an imprint of Times Mirror International Publishers Limited

Printed by Grafos S. A. Arte sobre papel, Barcelona, Spain.

ISBN 0 7234 17865

For full details of all Times Mirror International Publishers Limited titles, please write to Times Mirror International Publishers Limited, Lynton House, 7–12 Tavistock Square, London WC1H 9LB, England.

Contents

Foreword

The dental profession's current ability to elicit a so-called osseointegration response in virtually any edentulous site has profoundly changed prosthodontic practice. The era of maladaptive denture experience could very well be over, because both patients and dentists have already benefitted immeasurably from the technique. Much has been written about the osseointegration method, but this Atlas appears to be the first text intended for senior undergraduates and recently qualified dentists. As such, it is a welcome and superb contribution. It is well organised and provides a tidy, logical and step-by-step clinical approach, which is sensible and easy to follow. It is a compact and extremely well-illustrated treatise and actually ends up being more than a general introduction to the technique. It is an excellent review for experienced practitioners who have already worked in this field for some time.

Its format allows for the presentation of a rather complex procedure in a very attractive yet comprehensive manner. The material is beautifully integrated and I regard this atlas as a must for all dentists planning to use the osseointegration technique. The authors deserve the profession's gratitude for their outstanding contribution to dental education.

George A. Zarb
Toronto
Canada

Preface

Implant treatment has been one of the recent success stories of dentistry. Although the techniques have been practised for many years, until recently they proved to be largely unpredictable, often denigrated and with a dubious scientific foundation. Basic research has provided the clinician with a new and, in carefully selected patients, remarkably effective type of treatment. Inevitably this has acted as a spur to manufacturers, who are producing an ever-widening range of devices, while patients are beginning to request this type of treatment, sometimes with only a scanty and grossly optimistic understanding of what can be achieved. Much of the available information is technique or device-based. While the ability to master the skills of implant insertion and restoration is important, of far greater significance is the ability to set this form of treatment in a broader context. A basic understanding of the principles of the subject, coupled with treatment planning skills, will ultimately bring the greatest clinical benefits to our patients.

Today dentists may have their first contact with the topic as senior students or recent graduates undergoing further training, and it is for these groups that this book is principally intended. We hope that they will find it helpful.

Acknowledgments

We would like to thank the many clinical and technical colleagues who have helped us in the preparation of this book, reflecting the importance of teamwork in successful treatment with implants. We are especially grateful to the technical staff at both our institutions and, in particular, Mr Trevor Coward at Kings and Mr Cameron Malton at the Eastman. The staff of the Audio-Visual Departments have been most supportive in the preparation of studio views of our patients and macrophotographs of the many small components. Mr Richard Welfare, Dr David Davis and Mr Ken Hemmings have kindly loaned us pictures of some of their cases, and the companies associated with the Calcitek [C], Nobelpharma [N] and Steri-Oss [S] implant systems have kindly provided us with illustrations of their components for inclusion in the book. Thanks also to Mr Michael Gaukroger, who undertook the work featured on pages 156–7. Above all, our secretaries, Hilary Ward and Liz Pier, have retained their good humour and space on their hard disks, in the face of an evolving text and tight deadlines. We thank them all.

John A. Hobkirk
Roger M. Watson

1. Principles of Osseointegration

Bone healing

Irrespective of the trigger-inducing injury to a bone, a similar series of healing events will ensue. Hence a fracture, the insertion of a bone graft or surgical intervention, such as drilling a hole for an oral implant, will produce a common response in the tissues. Possible intermediate fragments in the fracture do, in fact, resemble a free bone graft and even the incorporation of an implant will result in the obeying of similar rules with respect to the bone healing situation. This is on condition that the graft is of an autogenous origin so that it does not elicit an immunological response and that the implant materials (at least for the purpose of the discussion) may be regarded as totally inert. The purpose of this chapter is to formulate the general background to bone repair with some added comments on the slightly more complicated healing situation of the implant. With respect to incorporation of oral implants, the concept of osseointegration has had a profound influence which is why there is a need for discussion of the definitions of this term. Thereafter, the cellular background to osseointegration will be discussed, followed by comments on the six factors regarded as important control objects for a reliable bone anchorage of a foreign material. The chapter will end with some concluding remarks.

Definitions of osseointegration

Osseointegration is based on the idea of a stable bone anchorage of an oral implant in contrast to a soft-tissue anchorage of the same that is known to function poorly over long terms of follow-up. This may seem peculiar as the tooth itself is anchored in soft tissue. However, a tooth is attached with a highly differentiated periodontal ligament, in sharp contrast to the poorly organised soft-tissue attachment of an oral implant. In fact, soft-tissue of a scar-like type is what develops around foreign materials such as metals inserted in the oral cavity and no-one has so far been able to re-establish a true ligament around such implant replacements. In the past this type of soft-tissue attachment of oral implants was regarded as unavoidable, resulting in a gradual loosening of the inserted biomaterial. Brånemark and co-workers[6] were the first to suggest the possibility of a direct bone to metal anchorage that they later termed 'osseointegration' (**1.1**), a concept that today has been widely accepted in oral implantology as the outcome of osseointegrated implants has been documented to be excellent also over long periods of follow-up (Albrektsson & Sennerby[2]). However, attempts to define osseointegration based on histologic criteria have failed (**1.2**), and today the only acceptable definition seems to be based on a confirmed and maintained implant stability as suggested by Zarb & Albrektsson, 1991:

"Osseointegration is a process whereby clinically asymptomatic rigid fixation of alloplastic materials is achieved, and maintained, in bone during functional loading".

Cellular background to osseointegration

The conditions for a proper bone response to occur include the presence of adequate cells, an adequate nutrition to these cells and an adequate stimulus for bone repair. The adequate cells are differentiated bone cells (osteoblast, osteoclast and osteocyte) on the one hand and undifferentiated cells that may be stimulated in the direction of an osteogenic induction on the other (**1.3**). However, in reality bone healing is dependent not only on the recruitment of new bone tissue, but also on an appropriate amount of newly formed soft-tissue, including capillaries, to take but one example. **1.4** demonstrates the resultant sequence of reactions initiated by 'injury', a not very subtle but correct way of describing the stimulus for repair. Injury will sensitise cells as well as release particular growth factors that will act by stimulating these cells. Again, the inevitable trauma to bone at every surgical procedure involving that tissue will trigger not only the formation of new bone, but also the formation of various soft tissues. The balance between the different tissue elements involved in bone repair is influenced by mediators elicited from the cells. There are autocrine as well as paracrine control mechanisms[7]. This delicate balance may be easily disturbed by external influences, for instance movements that will turn the balance in favour of new soft tissue formation instead of bone. Other known circumstances that affect bone healing are, for instance, pH or O_2-saturation. That the adequate stimulus for bone repair is 'injury' should not lead to the false conclusion that more injury will result in a greater healing response; indeed, the opposite seems to be the case. Too much injury will result in permanent damage to the repair tissues and healing will not ensue. The research field of whatever healing signal that is triggered by the injury is a vast one and the details of the research on healing factors are beyond the scope of this presentation, not least because current research on various bone growth factors will probably change the scene dramatically. Recent reviews have been presented by Mohan & Baylink[10] and, with special reference to the periodontal healing situation, by Wirthlin[11]. In the case of bone healing, the adequate stimulus has been regarded by various authors as based on either a cell-to-cell contact, soluble matrix molecules or stress-generated electric potentials (1.5a–c). In the first case, the influence is centred on the cellular component of bone. Surviving or even dying bone cells are thought capable of eliciting a chemical signal that will influence adjacent undifferentiated cells to choose to become preosteoblasts. Healing signals will arise from surviving or dying soft-tissue cells to persuade the same undifferentiated mother cell to become a prefibroblast, that once made Hulth[8] formulate his bone healing theory based on 'competing healing factors'. The second school emphasises the ground substance rather than the cellular influence. Protein signals are being released from the matrix component of the injured bone and will then trigger the undifferentiated cells as summarised above. The bone inductive capacity of devitalised bone matrix has been demonstrated without any reasonable doubts. The currently most well-known research group in the field of matrix influence is the Bone Induction School at Urist in Los Angeles. Thirdly, there may be stress-generated electric signals that trigger the healing response, as postulated by yet other well-known researchers such as Brighton and Bassett. In reality, of course, all three theories may be correct.

Factors of importance to ensure a reliable bone anchorage of an implanted device

In most cases whenever an implant is inserted in bone, healing will ensue dependent on the conditions listed above – adequate cells, nutrition to these cells and adequate stimuli for repair. However, bone tissue is different from soft-tissue in some aspects. In the first place bone will, at least under ideal conditions, heal without any scar formation due to ongoing creeping substitution (1.6) that will gradually replace the bone with newly formed hard tissue. Secondly, even if the repair process is disturbed so that no (or very little) healing ensues, the dead bone may (like a dead branch of a tree) still be capable of carrying some loads and thereby contribute to function. This may in clinical practice be the case in many hip and knee arthroplasties. Such replacements may tolerate the load put upon them by an elderly patient, but not the more heavy stress likely in young individuals where the results are much less good than with senior citizens. Only the third alternative, a dominant bone resorption will, if persistent, result in no function whatsoever (1.7). The delicate balance between bone formation and bone resorption may be exemplified through the known coupled function between bone cellular elements of opposing function such as osteoblasts and osteoclasts. Many authors claim that the one cell will need the other to be in an active state (1.8). This is further exemplified in the previously described creeping substitution process.

Even if osseointegrated implants have been documented to result in excellent long-term results, this does not necessarily imply that every implant system claimed to be dependent on osseointegration will result in an acceptable clinical outcome. On the contrary, there are several reasons for primary as well as secondary failure of osseointegration[4]. These failures may be attributed to an inadequate control of the six different factors known to be important for the establishment of a reliable, long-term osseous anchorage of an implanted device[3]. These factors are: (1) implant biocompatibility, (2) design characteristics, (3) surface characteristics, (4) the state of the host bed, (5) the surgical technique, and (6) the loading conditions. There is a need to control these factors more or less simultaneously to achieve the desirable goal of a direct bone anchorage. The focus of this presentation is to summarise the current opinion on the six factors. However, for full details, including references, the reader is referred to recent review papers on the subject[1,5].

Implant biocompatibility

With respect to metals, commercially pure (c.p.) titanium, niobium and possibly tantalum are known to be most well accepted in bone tissue. In the case of c.p. titanium, there is likewise a documented positive long-term function. The reason for the good acceptance of these metals does probably relate to the fact that they are covered with a very adherent, self-repairing oxide layer which has an excellent resistance to corrosion. Whereas the load-bearing capacity of c.p. titanium is sufficiently documented in the case of oral implants, there is less known about niobium in this aspect. Other metals such as different cobalt-chrome-molybdenum alloys and stainless steels have demonstrated less good take in the bone bed, but it is uncertain if this is valid for every possible such alloy and if it is a biocompatibility effect alone that is responsible for their less satisfactory incorporation into bone, compared with c.p.

titanium. A significantly impaired interfacial bone formation compared to c.p. titanium has been found with titanium-6aluminium-4vanadium alloy, prob-ably dependent on a less good biocompatibility of the alloy. One concern with metal alloys is that one alloy component may leak out in concentrations high enough to cause local or systemic side-effects. However, whether these and other differences between c.p. titanium on the one hand and various alloys on the other are of a practical, clinical importance or of only a theoretical one is uncertain, which is why the alloys have been placed in the yellow zone (**1.9**). In the red zone, definitely, are metals such as copper and silver that are known to result in a permanent soft-tissue attachment because of poor biocompatibility. Ceramics such as the calcium phosphate hydroxyapatite (HA) should definitely be in the green zone, whereas various types of aluminium oxides are in the yellow region (**1.9**), due to insufficient documentation. With respect to HA, the available literature points to at least a short-term (<10 weeks) enhanced interfacial bone formation in comparison to various reference metals. This represents a potential clinical benefit of HA, whereas the risk for coat loosening with subsequent problems represents a potential risk (**1.10**).

Implant design

There is, at present, sufficient long-term docu-mentation only on threaded types of oral implants that have been demonstrated to function for decades without clinical problems. However, unthreaded implants may function too, even if there is a total lack of positive documentation with respect to bone saucerisation, a problem that caused failure of many early types of oral implants. With currently used cylindrical implants, some 10 publications describe more severe bone resorption than would have been expected with certain screw designs[3]. It must be observed that there are other unthreaded implant designs than those depicted in **1.11**, that may give an excellent long-term clinical result, albeit undocumented at the time of writing this chapter.

Implant surface

With respect to the surface topography there is clear documentation that most smooth surfaces do not result in an acceptable bone cell adhesion. Such implants do therefore end up as being anchored in soft tissue despite the material used . Clinical failure would be prone to occur. Some microirregularities seem to be necessary for a proper cellular adhesion even if the optimal surface topography remains to be described. With

a gradual increase of the surface topographical irregularities, problems due to an increased ionic leakage are prone to occur. With plasma-sprayed titanium surfaces for instance, more than 1600 ppm titanium has been reported in implant-adjacent haversian systems, probably resulting in an impairment of osteogenesis (**1.12**).

Another surface parameter is the energy state where a high surface energy has been regarded as positive for implant take due to an alleged, improved cellular attachment. One practical way of increasing the surface energy is the use of glow discharge (plasma cleaning). However, published reports have not been able to confirm the superiority of so artificially enhanced implant energy levels. One reason for this lack of confirmation of the surface energy hypothesis could be that the increased surface energy will disappear immediately when the implant makes in contact with the host tissues.

In conclusion, there is little doubt that new research efforts will be necessary to learn more about the implant surface and its importance for osseointegration[9].

State of the host bed

If available, the ideal host bed is healthy and with an adequate bone stock. However, in the clinical reality, the host bed may suffer from previous irradiation, ridge height resorption and osteoporosis, to mention some undesirable states for implantation (**1.13**). Previous irradiation need not be an absolute contraindication for the insertion of oral implants. However, it is preferrable that some delay is allowed before an implant is inserted into a previously irradiated bed. Furthermore, some 10–15% poorer clinical results must be anticipated after a therapeutical dose of irradiation. The explan-ation for less satisfactory clinical outcome found in irradiated beds could be vascular damage, at least in part. One attempt to increase the healing conditions in a previously irradiated bed is by using hyperbaric oxygen, as a low oxygen tension definitely has negative effects on tissue repair. This is further verified by the finding that heavy smoking, causing among other things a local oral vasoconstriction, is one factor that will lower the expected outcome of an implantation procedure.

Other common clinical host bed problems involve osteoporosis and resorbed alveolar ridges. Such clinical states may constitute an indication for ridge augmentation with bone grafts. However, present clinical techniques for bone grafting are under debate and it appears that a 5-year success of oral implants in the 75% range is a realistic outcome after most such procedures. This figure is slightly alarming seen against the fact that, at least in the maxilla, 10–20% of an average edentulous population may be in need of a bone graft to improve the host bed and allow for the insertion of implants. On the contrary, if the bone quality and quantity in the maxilla is controlled, the expected outcome of an oral implantation procedure is similar to that of the mandible.

Surgical technique

If too violent a surgical technique is used, frictional heat will cause a temperature rise in the bone and the cells that should be responsible for bone repair will be destroyed. Bone tissue is more sensitive to heat than previously believed. In the past the critical temperature was regarded to be in the 56°C range, as this temperature will cause denaturation of one of the bone enzymes, alkaline phosphatase. However, the critical time/temperature relationship for bone tissue necrosis is around 47°C applied for one minute. At a temperature of 50°C applied for more than one minute we are coming close to a critical level where bone repair becomes severely and permanently disturbed. This critical temperature should be seen against observed frictional heat at surgical interventions. In the orthopaedic field, despite adequate cooling, temperatures of 90°C have been measured. High drilling temperatures in the dental field are to be expected when drilling, particularly in the dense mandible. Figure **1.14** demonstrates the importance of using well sharpened drills, slow drill speeds, a graded series of drills (avoid making, for instance, a 4 mm hole in one step) and adequate cooling. By using such a controlled technique it has been demonstrated in clinical studies that overheating may be totally avoided. The mechanical injury will of course remain and is quite sufficient to trigger a proper healing response.

Another surgical parameter of relevance is the power used at implant insertion. Too strong a hand will result in bone tension and a resorption response will be stimulated. This means that the holding power of the implant will fall to dangerous levels after a strong insertion torque. A moderate power at the screwing home of an implant is therefore recommended. With other implant designs there may be a need for impaction of the implant at insertion and other rules may apply.

Loading conditions

From histological investigations of animal as well as human implants we know that, irrespective of control of surgical trauma and other relevant parameters, the implant will, in the early remodelling phase, be surrounded by soft tissue. This means that some weeks after implant insertion it will be particularly sensitive to loading that results in movements, as movement will stimulate more soft-tissue formation, leading eventually to a permanent soft-tissue anchorage. In essence, the situation is similar to that of a fracture (**1.15**). Loading of an unstabilised fracture will result in soft tissue healing and poor function, whereas stabilisation with plates or Plaster of Paris will ensure a satisfying rigidity leading to bone healing of the fracture. The case of an implant (**1.16**) is, in principle, very similar. Premature loading will lead to soft-tissue anchorage and poor long-term function, whereas postponing the loading by using a two-stage surgery will result in bone healing and positive long-term function. The length of time loading should be avoided is dependent on the implantation site as well as on the the bone bed quality. Furthermore, there may be cases where an almost immediate loading would not disturb the bone-healing response, but in general loading must be controlled if osseointegration is to occur. Brånemark with his controlled implant system advocated the use of a 3-month loading delay in the mandible and a 4–6 month delay in the healthy maxilla where the bone is, as a rule, more cancellous in character. However, these precise unloaded times are empirically based and to the knowledge of the author there are no published studies comparing different unloaded periods and relating this to implant success. Furthermore, from a bone biologic point of view a more suitable design would be to have the implant unloaded and then gradually increase the load in the manner of the Sarmiento technique for functional braces in fracture healing. The problem in the case of oral implants is how properly to define to the patient how a gradual increase of load should be controlled; a complicated task not the least since the appropriate loading pattern also depends on individual patient factors.

Concluding remarks

To this day the use of poorly controlled techniques in oral implantology continues and the lack of clinical data to back up many types of oral implants is alarming. Osseointegration has meant a clinical breakthrough in a discipline, oral implantology, previously regarded as *non lege artis*. A scientific approach to any clinical treatment calls not only for well controlled implantation procedures but also for an honest and meticulous reporting of clinical data. Any clinical routine usage of untested procedures or oral implant designs should be avoided until sufficient documentation is available and reported over a minimum of 5 years of follow-up.

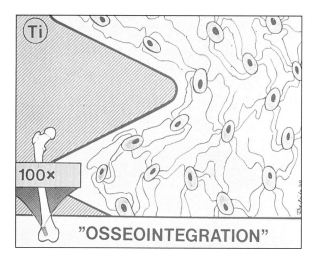

1.1 Osseointegration. Osseointegration is a term originally coined by Brånemark who was of the opinion that bone tissue embedded the implant more or less totally, resulting in a stable interface under clinical loading.

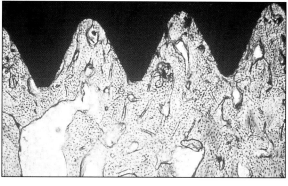

1.2 In the biologic reality there is no evidence of a complete bone to implant contact, but there is more or less soft tissue. Nevertheless, at the light microscopic level of resolution there is adequate evidence for osseointegration, even if there is no consensus to a histologically based definition of the term.

1.3 Adequate cells. The adequate cells for bone tissue repair are the differentiated bone cells such as the bone-forming osteoblast and the osteocyte and the bone-resorbing osteoclast. New osteoblasts are recruited from primitive mesenchymal cells that, with a proper stimulus, will become induced in osteogenic direction. The same undifferentiated mesenchymal cell may, with another stimulus, instead develop into a soft-tissue fibroblast.

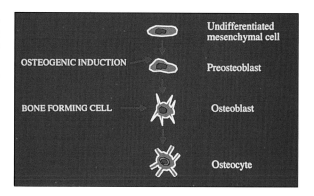

1.4 Phases of healing. One way of looking at the initiation of bone repair is to regard 'injury' as the initiating mechanism. Injury is known to act as a releasing stimulus for various growth factors as well as to sensitise various cell types (top). The second healing phase at a few weeks after injury has been termed the granulation stage. At this time new local connective tissue, new capillaries and supportive tissue appear, whereas an abundant new bone formation is generally not seen until the next healing stage (middle). In the so-called Callus phase of bone healing, there has been a delicate balance established among the several tissues that proliferate in the case of a bone injury. Information between the different cellular subgroups is maintained via chemical signals – mediators. Outer influence may disturb the balance, leading to poor bone healing (bottom).

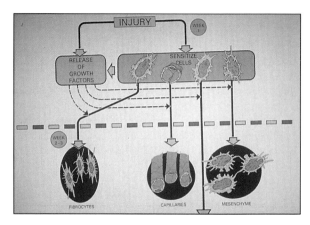

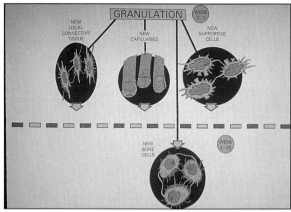

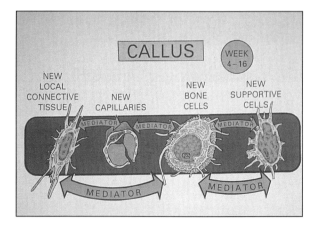

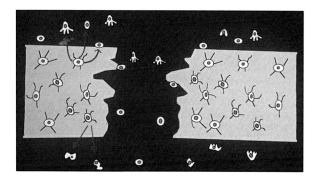

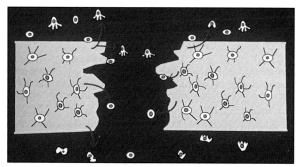

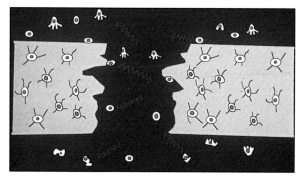

1.5 Adequate stimulus for bone repair. 'Injury' is not a very subtle way of describing the proper stimulus for bone repair. According to one school, there is a cell-to-cell contact as surviving or maybe dying cells in the fracture area will send out chemical signals to adjacent undifferentiated cells to start differentiation into new cellular lines (top). Another school emphasises instead the matrix contribution. Soluble matrix molecules leak out from the injured bone and those molecules are the trigger mechanism for the undifferentiated cells (middle). Some other investigators claim that the main stimulus for repair is derived from piezoelectric signals elicited by the movements of the fracture ends. Most certainly, these three theories need not stand in opposition to one another but may all be correct. Even if the example has been referring to fracture healing, similar rules apply to implant incorporation (bottom).

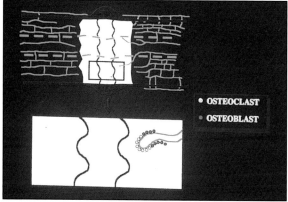

1.6 Creeping substitution. Cortical bone repair is known to occur through a process called creeping substitution. Vessels penetrate the necrotic border zone of the fracture according to the pathway of least resistance. Osteoclasts resorb the necrotic bone and osteoblasts form new bone around the vessel. As many such vessels penetrate the bone growing in different directions, the new bone laid down around the various vessels will be of an unordered nature in relation to the surrounding ordered bone. With time, however, continuing creeping substitution with vessels gradually growing in a more straight and ordered fashion will result in remodelling of the bone in the fracture area so that, in the end, the fracture will heal completely without any scar formation, at least in the theoretically ideal situation.

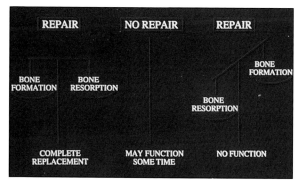

1.7 Bone tissue reactions to injury. Bone tissue reaction to injury can be described as a lever balance with the ideal resulting in a complete replacement situation. The contrast is represented by the persistent dominance of bone resorption and replacement with soft tissue, seen for instance when there is continuous movement in the fracture ends when no function will ensue. In some clinical cases, there is little or no healing which may result in some function, as also dead bone (like the dead branch of a tree) may carry some loads.

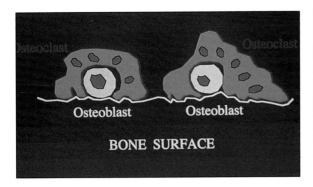

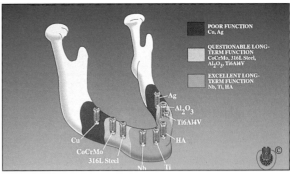

1.8 Osteoclast/osteoblast coupled function. Cells of opposing function such as the osteoblast (bone-forming) and the osteoclast (bone-resorbing) demonstrate a coupled function so that the activity of the one cell is dependent on the presence of the other. One example of coupled function is represented by the creeping substitution process.

1.9 Implant biocompatibility. Materials that have been demonstrated as most tolerant to bone tissue are exemplified by commercially pure titanium and niobium and hydroxyapatite (HA) in the green region of the mandible. Other materials, such as stainless steel, cobalt chrome molybdenum alloys, aluminium oxides and titanium-6aluminium-4vanadium alloys are more questionable with respect to documented long-term function and are therefore found in the yellow region. In the red region are clearly unsuitable metals such as copper and silver. It is understood that if new documentation so indicates then materials may be moved, for instance, from the yellow to the green zone.

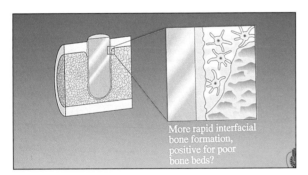

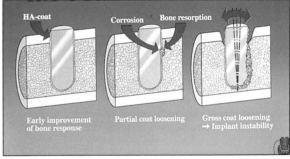

1.10 HA-coated implants. The great advantage with HA is the reported indications of this material eliciting a more rapid bone response than uncoated metals such as c.p. titanium. This may be of clear advantage, particularly in bone beds of an assumed poor repair capability (left). The risk associated with HA is predominantly that of coat loosening, however unknown in frequency, subsequent bone saucerisation and other problems (right).

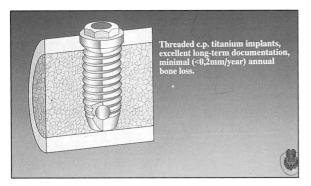

Threaded c.p. titanium implants, excellent long-term documentation, minimal (<0,2mm/year) annual bone loss.

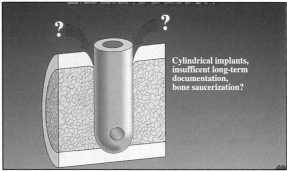

Cylindrical implants, insufficent long-term documentation, bone saucerization?

1.11 Implant design. The threaded implant design has been thoroughly documented over long period of follow-up (left). In the case of cylindrical designs, there is no doubt that several different types of cylinders have been found possible to anchor in bone, but long-term documentation is lacking. Such long-term documentation must be gathered to find out whether several reports of bone saucerisation adjacent to cylindrical implants represent the exceptions or the rule, a question that cannot be reliably answered without a proper documentation over at least 5 years of follow-up (right).

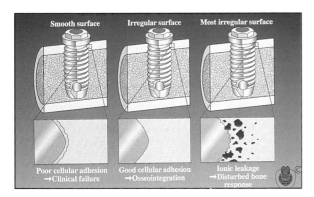

Smooth surface | Irregular surface | Most irregular surface

Poor cellular adhesion →Clinical failure | Good cellular adhesion →Osseointegration | Ionic leakage →Disturbed bone response

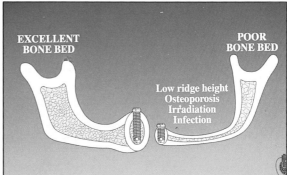

EXCELLENT BONE BED

POOR BONE BED

Low ridge height Osteoporosis Irradiation Infection

1.12 Implant surface. The ideal implant surface remains to be described. It is, however, known that polished surfaces are unsuitable for bone implantation. Surface irregularities seem necessary for cellular attachment. Most irregular surfaces are negative for osseointegration for geometric reasons as well as with respect to the increased risk of long-term problems due to ionic leakage that is increased with increased tissue–metal contact area. However, no-one has been able to describe properly the size of the greatest recommended surface irregularities, probably because of methodological shortcomings. In addition, there are other surface parameters of potential importance such as the level of surface energy.

1.13 State of the host bed. The excellent bone bed is healthy and with an adequate amount and quality of bone. The poor bone bed suffers from low ridge height, osteoporosis, previous irradiation and infection, all conditions that by themselves may represent at least relative contraindications for routine insertion of implants other than in university clinics.

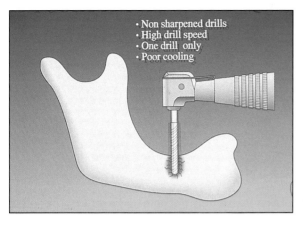

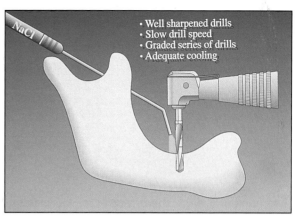

1.14 Surgical technique. A poor surgical technique results in healing problems and can be due to blunt drills, high drill speed or poor cooling (left). Optimal surgery is achieved by control of these factors and by the use of a graded series of drills instead of the initial use of the largest size (right).

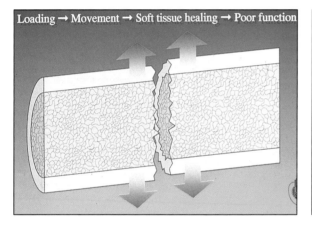

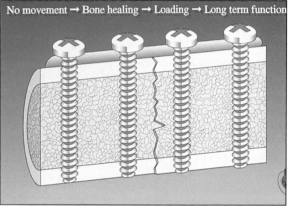

1.15 Fracture treatment. The fracture that is allowed free, unrestricted movements will show poor or no bone healing (left). Stabilisation of fractures with Plaster of Paris or plates will minimise movement and the chances of proper bone healing are thus clearly increased (right).

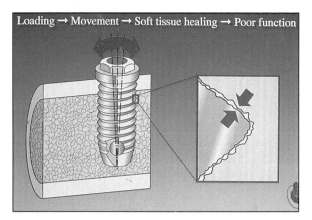

Loading → Movement → Soft tissue healing → Poor function

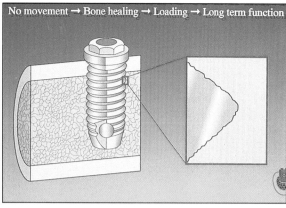

No movement → Bone healing → Loading → Long term function

1.16 Loading of implant. As the bone implant inevitably will be surrounded by soft tissue during the early healing stages, loading then will result in movement with a subsequent soft-tissue healing and poor function (left). Premature movement of the implant is assured by postponing loading until the foreign material has had time to become properly anchored in bone, a process that takes about 3 months in the mandible. Long-term function is now possible (right).

2. Anatomical Considerations

Introduction

The successful use of endosseous implants involves the creation and maintenance of a load-bearing bone–implant interface stabilising a suitable prosthesis. This prosthesis must meet the patient's requirements in terms of function and appearance, whilst contributing to the long-term stability of the implant–host interface on which the ultimate success of the treatment depends. Two factors are important in maintenance of the interface: plaque control and force transmission. Facilitation of cleansing by the patient of the superstructure and the intra-oral implant components is a major design objective, yet it is one that often conflicts with aesthetic demands. This is because the position of the implants is limited by the bony envelope within which they must be contained. The occlusal and buccal or labial aspects of the implant superstructure may need to be placed some distance from the edentulous ridges if optimum appearance, and sometimes masticatory function, are to be produced. The problems of linking artificial teeth placed in the positions of their natural predecessors with implants housed in the residual alveolar ridge are demonstrated in the series of figures from **2.1** to **2.7**.

Since the implant–bone interface is strain-sensitive, consideration must be given to the manner in which occlusal loads may be transmitted to the implant. This will be influenced by the physical relationship of the occlusal surface of the superstructure to the underlying implants. Where they are essentially in the same vertical axis then the patterns of load transmission will be very different to those where cantilevering exists. This results in torquing forces that are thought to be particularly hazardous to osseointegrated interfaces. It should be remembered that cantilevering can occur both bucco-lingually and antero-posteriorly.

Some features of the design of an implant superstructure are specifically related to its method of support, others will reflect principles of extension and contour which are equally relevant to the design of a fixed bridge, partial denture saddle or complete denture. These relate principally to the different methods of stabilising fixed and removable appliances, and the design features that must be incorporated into a fixed appliance to simplify oral hygiene. Thus the extent of a fixed appliance is limited by these considerations, whilst a removable appliance may need greater extension to restore function and provide adequate support.

If appropriate patients are to be selected for implant treatment then it is essential that the clinician has a clear understanding of the anatomy of those structures that have been lost, and those that remain. It is on the replacement of the former, using devices placed in the latter, that successful implant treatment depends.

Just as the foundation for a building must reflect its design and the shape and properties of the underlying ground, so must implant positioning be linked not only to tissue anatomy but also to superstructure design.

As implants are used solely to provide a method of mechanical linkage to the facial skeleton, the anatomy of the bones is central to this consideration. The soft tissues are also important in this context as they delineate much of the prosthesis space, and may provide some support for an overdenture.

The principal factors that need to be considered are:

- The prosthesis space. This is analogous to the denture space.
- The size and shape of the alveolar ridge and underlying bone.
- The structure of the bone within the jaw.
- The position of structures within or next to the ridge that might influence surgical procedures.
- The contours of the soft tissues overlying the alveolar ridge.
- The nature of the soft tissues overlying the alveolar ridge.

Assessment techniques

Methods of assessment are based on clinical observation and records for the determination of the prosthesis space and to a certain extent bone contours, supplemented by radiographic techniques.

The prosthesis space may be evaluated by clinical examination including consideration of the existing prosthesis, palpation and direct measurement, for example with callipers. Study casts mounted in the intercuspal position, or the desired relationship in edentulous patients, can provide much information as to the probable position of the final prostheses and their relationships with the alveolar ridges. This is often helped by the construction of trial appliances and the production of overcasts. These matters are considered in more detail in Chapter 4.

Radiographic techniques that may be utilised include intra-oral views, including those with peri-apical film, preferably using a long-cone technique to minimise distortion. Other intra-oral views of value are true occlusal films of the anterior mandible. Tomograms of various types, of which the OPT is the most common, are particularly helpful, although this view is subject to considerable distortion and must be used with caution (**2.4**). Where it is contemplated that implants may be inserted in the anterior mandible then a lateral skull radiograph may prove useful as it provides in effect a mid-line sagittal section of the jaw (**4.38**). Whilst computerised tomograms (CAT scans) of the jaws are expensive, they are invaluable in determining with considerable precision the amount of bone available at potential implant sites, and are thus useful where this is limited. **2.8–2.11**, **2.13** and **2.14** show CAT scans of the edentulous skull in **2.2**, whilst those in **2.24** and **2.25** show the relatively small amount of bone that exists in the apparently ample edentulous ridge in the patient in **2.22** and **2.23**.

The prosthesis space

This space is determined by the relationship of the edentulous alveolar ridge to the adjacent and opposing teeth or edentulous ridge and the surrounding soft tissues. These relationships are of significance both at rest and in function and control the potential size and position of the superstructure, particularly where it replaces missing soft tissues or is extensive. The space is rarely entirely evident on examination, as following loss of the teeth and their supporting structures the surrounding soft tissues tend to collapse inwards leaving a small space. Thus, room for the prosthesis must be created by tissue displacement. The space is also dynamic in nature, being partly defined by patterns of muscular activity, which change to maximise function following loss of the teeth. Many patients, particularly elderly persons who have reduced learning abilities, may be unable to learn the necessary new skills to use a removable prosthesis.

The prosthesis space has both vertical and horizontal components. Vertical separation of the jaws at rest, and therefore the room for the freeway space and the natural teeth or their artificial successors, are important factors in all restorative dentistry, but especially in implant treatment. The vertical separation of the jaws at rest must accommodate the freeway space, the implant superstructure, clearance below the prosthesis to allow for cleaning by the patient, and the opposing natural or artificial dentition (**2.21**). Over-eruption of opposing natural teeth, an altered rest position, enlargement of the edentulous ridges and an unusually large freeway space can all lead to problems.

The vertical dimension of the face is influenced in rest by muscle activity and the elasticity of the peri-oral tissues and in function by the natural teeth, if any. Where these have been lost, become excessively worn or been inadequately replaced, then an altered and sometimes abnormally large freeway space or inter-occlusal clearance may exist. A patient's ability to tolerate a change in this will have implications for the implant superstructure, be it fixed or removable, and must be recognised before implant placement.

Following the loss of the teeth and inevitable alveolar resorption, the soft tissues will tend to encroach upon the space that they formerly occupied. As a result the tongue spreads laterally and the cheeks collapse inwards producing the well recognised effects of tooth loss on facial appearance. Restoration of this lost space, which must be recaptured from the soft tissues by the prosthesis, is partly dependent upon their elasticity and partly upon the patient's ability to adapt to change. It must therefore be recognised that the dynamic aspects of the denture space are extremely important. The extent to which the space may be restored successfully is dependent upon the patient's adaptability, desire for a natural appearance and the prosthetist's skills. Whilst a detailed consideration of this topic is outside the scope of this book, it is referred to in Chapter 4. It is important to recognise that any implant-stabilised prosthesis must be in harmony with its environment, and that implants should not be used to stabilise prostheses that are inherently inadequate. Failure to do so can lead to marked discomfort, problems with cheek and tongue biting, and impaired speech.

Faced with a requirement to replace missing teeth and supporting tissues, there are several anatomical landmarks that may be employed as guides. These are usually known as biometric guides. They include the incisive papilla, the renant of the maxillary palatal gingival margin, the retromolar pads, the alar-tragal line, and the position of the lips and their relationships. These guides are particularly relevant to the design of overdentures; however, it is important to recognise that they are but guides and that the ultimate arbiter of the prosthesis space must be the functional activities of the soft tissues.

The incisive papilla

This structure normally lies palatal to the maxillary central incisors with its mid-point some 10 mm palatal to their labial aspect. Following loss of the teeth, labial alveolar resorption results in the papilla coming to lie slightly more labially and thus the anterior aspect of the incisors should usually be some 10 mm anterior to its palatal margin.

The remnant of the palatal gingival margin

Watt has shown that, in the edentulous patient, it is possible to identify a thin fibrous band near the crest of the alveolar ridge. This represents the remnant of the palatal gingival margin, from which measurements can be taken to aid in the positioning of artificial teeth if it is desired to place these in the positions of their natural predecessors. Figure **6.54** demonstrates the cantilevering which was necessary to bring the artificial teeth on a maxillary implant-stabilised fixed-bridge prosthesis into occlusion with a dentate lower jaw.

The retromolar pads

These structures consist of aggregations of fibrous tissue overlaid with mucosa and represent the distal aspect of the dental arch. It is unusual for them to lie much lower than the occlusal plane. A useful guide to the positioning of the lingual cusps of the artificial mandibular posterior teeth is that they should lie within a triangle bounded by the tip of the canine tooth and the buccal and lingual margins of the retromolar pad.

The retromolar pads are often also used to delineate the distal border of a lower denture; however, this is better achieved functionally if maximum extension is to be achieved, since the underlying buccinator and temporalis muscles have variable form and patterns of activity. The distal fibres of the buccinator muscle sweep over the mandible from its lateral aspect to be inserted into the pterygomandibular raphe on its medial aspect, whilst deeper the fibres of the temporalis muscle run vertically to be inserted into the anterior aspect of the ramus.

The alar-tragal line

The alar-tragal line provides a convenient guide to antero-posterior orientation of the maxillary occlusal plane with which it is normally parallel.

The position of the lips and their relationships

The contours of the lips can provide a useful, although somewhat subjective, guide to the positioning of anterior teeth when designing a prosthesis as, whilst the collapse following the loss of teeth is well recognised, the desired contour is less easily defined. The principal contours of value are the naso-labial angle, the angle between the left and right contours of the upper lip when viewed from below, and the contact between the edges of the upper incisors and the lower lip at rest, which should be near the junction of the matt and glossy mucosa.

The size and shape of the alveolar ridge

The size and shape of the alveolar ridge following the loss of the teeth are of particular concern to the dentist as they govern the feasibility of inserting endosseous implants and their relationship to an overlying prosthesis.

Following the loss of natural teeth, resorption of the alveolar bone inevitably occurs, although at an exponentially reducing rate, and thus a potential space comes to exist between the anatomically correct positions of the artificial teeth and the edentulous ridge.

In the mandible alveolar resorption initially reduces the height of the anterior ridge at a rate typically 4 times that in the maxilla, whilst resorption occurs more rapidly on the labial aspect of the ridge anteriorly, resulting in its crest tending to move lingually. Posteriorly resorption is greater from the lingual aspect, and thus the alveolar ridge becomes progressively lower, wider distally, and displaced towards the tongue anteriorly.

In the maxilla, in addition to reduction in the height of the crest of the ridge, there is also resorption from the buccal and labial aspects at a rate which is greater than palatally so that the crest of the ridge effectively moves inwards. As dental implants have to be placed in the ridge it becomes necessary to cantilever any superstructure placed upon them.

The sectioned casts shown in **2.15–2.20** show the effect of resorption on the relationships of the ridges in the sagittal planes in patients with Class I, II and III apical base relationships.

In **2.15–2.17** the changes in the relationship of the anterior ridges in a patient with a Class I type of incisor relationship are shown. It will be noted that the effects of loss of maxillary teeth are particularly severe in terms of the cantilevering which becomes necessary to provide an acceptable occlusion.

The sections shown in **2.18** and **2.19** show the situation for patients with a Class II apical base relationship and a Class II division 2 incisor pattern. In the anterior region in the Class II2 case (**2.19**) the problems of restoring the occlusion with an implant-stabilised prosthesis are evident.

Figure **2.20** shows the effects of tooth loss where

the patient has a mild Class III type of apical base relationship, which tends to exacerbate the problems of using maxillary implants opposed by a dentate lower jaw.

The size of the alveolar ridge is of significance in that it determines the feasibility of placing an implant within the bone, as there are manufacturer-determined restrictions on the minimum width of device available and practical restraints on the minimum length of implant which it is appropriate to use. Most manufacturers produce implants with diameters of the order of 3.5–4.0 mm, although there are some available which are only 2.5 mm in diameter (see also Chapter 3). As it is necessary to allow a space of at least 1 mm around the implant, the minimum ridge thickness which can be normally utilised is of the order of 6–7 mm. This may present problems in either jaw, although it is more difficult to manage in the maxilla and posteriorly in the mandible. The CAT scan in **2.11** shows the thin bony crest which may remain on the mandibular basal bone after resorption. This is usually too narrow to house an implant and would thus have to be completely removed to allow successful fixture insertion. The effects of attempting to insert an implant in this situation without ridge reduction are shown in **2.34**.

Whilst it is often possible to insert implants into the mandibular basal bone anteriorly even where the jaw is relatively shallow, posteriorly, the presence of the mandibular canal precludes this unless the canal is placed lateral to the required position for the implants (**2.31**).

Whilst a similar pattern of resorption may be seen in the maxilla, labio-palatal thinning of the bone is often less severe, but may be enough to prevent inserting an implant. This is particularly significant in the upper jaw where resorption of the alveolar bone usually reveals a paucity of basal bone and the proximity of the nose and para-nasal sinuses to the residual alveolar ridges as shown in **2.14**. Because the prognosis of implants placed in the maxilla is related markedly to their length and 10 mm is usually considered to be the minimum which it is appropriate to use, many patients are precluded from this type of treatment. The CAT scans in **2.13** and **2.14** show the pattern of resorption which has occurred in the skull and the almost total obliteration of the maxillary alveolar bone is evident.

In addition to loss of height and width, a variation in the pattern of resorption of the alveolar ridge can result in a constriction below its crest which is hidden by the overlying soft tissues. This precludes placing implants within the ridge without

an augmentation procedure but may not be evident without very careful clinical examination or the use of specific radiographic views.

The orientation of the ridge

The orientation of the alveolar ridge is of special importance where its dimensions are restricted and where an angulated implant superstructure cannot be employed. In these situations the orientation of the superstructure inevitably then follows that dictated by the ridge contours, as it is neither possible to position the implants in the ridge more favourably or to utilise a different axis for the implant superstructure to that of the intra-bony component.

Where a patient has an Angles Class II$_1$ or II$_2$ incisor relationship, then the ridge orientation and the difficulties of placing a superstructure may prevent implant treatment (**2.19**, **2.20**).

The structure of the bone within the ridge

Successful osseointegration is dependent on an initial close unstressed contact between an implant and minimally traumatised bone. **2.26–2.29** demonstrate some examples of the patterns of bone which may be found within the jaws. These depict different amounts of bone in the cortex and medulla and, whilst it is possible to classify different combinations in some detail, the situation may not always be readily apparent in a clinical radiograph and usually varies from site to site in the jaw. This topic is considered in more detail in Chapter 4. Furthermore, the decision as to whether to treat a particular patient with implants is dependent on many factors, of which the bone pattern is but one. There are, however, a number of general principles which may be applied.

Bone which is dense and highly mineralised is difficult to prepare surgically and more likely to suffer thermal trauma during the procedure; however, it is more favourable from the viewpoint of achieving osseointegration.

Bone with a thick dense cortex but little cancellous bone can provide good implant fixation provided that it is possible to secure the implant in both cortices.

Situations where there is a thinner cortex in combination with dense cancellous bone will aid osseointegration. On the other hand bone with a thin cortex and little cancellous material internally may make initial fixation of the implant difficult and prejudice the long-term prognosis of the treatment both in terms of initial osseointegration and the subsequent load-bearing ability of the interface.

Structures of significance in implant placement

There are some structures adjacent to and within the jaws which are potentially of importance in using endosseous implants either because they may influence surgical procedures or because they place restrictions on the size of implants which may be used. The following are of particular note.

The mandibular canal

This runs in a curved path from the mandibular foramen to the mental foramen and contains the mandibular nerve and its associated artery and vein. Whilst the canal lies considerably below the alveolar crest in the dentate patient, following severe alveolar resorption it can come to lie very close to the crest of the ridge as shown in the OPT radiograph in **2.4**. As a result it often restricts the use of implants distal to the mental foramina. It should however be remembered that the canal does not always lie directly below the crest of the residual alveolar ridge but may be placed either lingually or buccally to it, and it is therefore sometimes possible to insert the implant lateral to the neurovascular bundle. This needs to be confirmed by tomography prior to surgery.

The floor of the mouth

The body of the mandible posteriorly may be relatively flat on its upper surface; however, its cross-section posteriorly is characterised by greater height buccally (**2.32**), and thus whilst it appears to be of adequate depth for implant insertion on an OPT radiograph, this may not be the case. As a result devices placed too far lingually can involve the floor of the mouth.

The nose and para-nasal sinuses

The CAT scan views of the edentulous skull in **2.13** and **2.14** demonstrate the extensive pneumatisation of the maxillae which can occur in the edentulous patient and which limit implant placement. Whilst it is possible to place additional bone below the mucosal lining of the maxillary sinuses or to extend the crest of the ridge with transplanted bone these techniques are inevitably less certain than where extensive bone already exists. The nose can limit placement of implants anteriorly as its floor may come to lie close to the crest of the residual alveolar ridge, and in extreme cases all alveolar bone may be resorbed anteriorly so that the oral and nasal mucosa are contiguous.

Muscle attachments

The prosthesis space is limited by the muscles which are attached to the mandible. Buccally and labially these are the buccinator and, anteriorly, the muscles of facial expression inserted into the lips, whilst the overlying masseter muscles also impinge on the space. Lingually the mylohyoid, palatoglossus, genioglossus, hyoglossus and superior constructor muscles, together with the pterygomandibular raphe, all influence the room available for the prosthesis. These muscles are of significance in appliance design, particularly where an implant-stabilised complete denture is utilised, as in function they determine its dimensions, being unfavourably related to the superior surface of the resorbed mandible or ridge.

Following resorption of the alveolar bone, the buccinator and its associated muscles may come to be inserted close to the crest of the ridge. They may then benefit from repositioning so as to extend the potential denture-bearing area and reduce muscle pull on the soft tissues surrounding the implants when they are exposed.

The contours of the soft tissues overlying the alveolar ridge

The soft tissues overlying the ridge are of considerable importance both from the surgical viewpoint and also subsequent to implant placement as they form the cuff around the abutments. Excessively mobile tissue can create problems either by being repeatedly tugged around the implant or by pulling against the superstructure, leading to inflammation and hyperplasia. Repositioning of the tissues may be necessary prior to implant placement if a more appropriate site cannot be utilised.

The physical properties of oral tissues

Implants are used to provide a relatively rigid and predictable method of transmitting intra-oral forces from a prosthesis to the facial skeleton. However, there are occasions when it may be necessary or desirable to obtain some support for an implant superstructure from either the mucoperiosteum or an adjacent tooth. In these circumstances the mechanical properties of the various force-transmitting systems which are being used must be borne in mind.

The implant–bone interface has been shown to be largely elastic and relatively rigid compared with a natural tooth, whilst the periodontal ligament demonstrates visco-elastic properties and allows displacements in function of the order of 50–100 µm. The dissimilarity in the intrusion stiffness of an implant and the mucoperiosteum is even greater as the latter will typically displace by 0.5–1.0 mm under a complete denture in function. These disparities must be allowed for in implant design and superstructure fabrication, and at least one implant system incorporates a flexible component intended to reduce stress concentration in the system.

It should also be remembered that, despite the comforting solidity of a dental cast, it has been demonstrated that the mandible flexes in function and, whilst this is a complex phenomenon, it is known that approximation and separation of the order of 0.5 mm may occur across the mid-line in the molar region. The significance of this in implant treatment is not known. However, bending forces applied to the mandible distal to the implants in the anterior segment may induce a variety of effects both around loaded implants and remote from them.

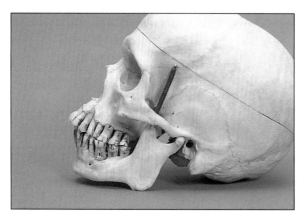

2.1 This dentate skull demonstrates the patterns of bone resorption associated with progressive loss of periodontal tissue.

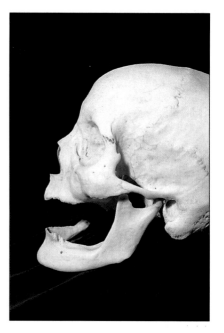

2.2 An edentulous skull showing the marked loss of alveolar bone. Reconstruction with an implant-stabilised prosthesis can present considerable difficulties for both the surgeon and the prosthodontist.

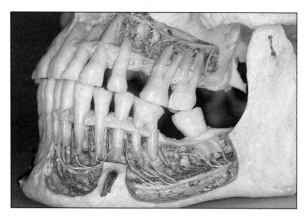

2.3 This prepared dentate skull shows the extent of the supporting tissues in the healthy adult.

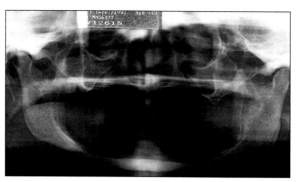

2.4 Considerable amounts of alveolar bone may be lost in the patient who has been edentulous for a considerable period. Compare the position of the mental foramina and mandibular canals with those in 2.3.

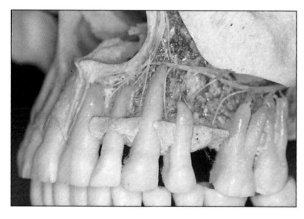

2.5 Whilst there is a considerable amount of bone around the canine and first premolar teeth in the maxilla, the apices of the incisor roots lie relatively close to the floor of the nose.

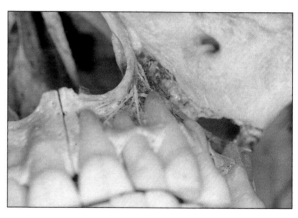

2.6 The roots of the molars lie close to the maxillary antrum which can be seen through a prepared hole adjacent to the apex of 26.

2.7 The amount of alveolar bone in the premaxilla, when viewed in sagittal section, is relatively restricted from the viewpoint of implant insertion.

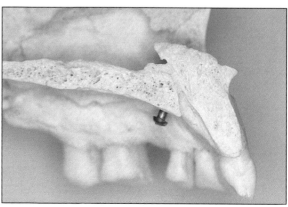

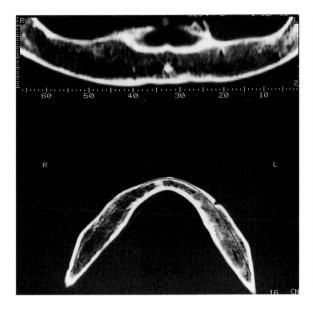

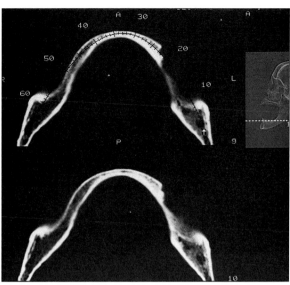

2.9 These CAT scan slices have been taken slightly below the top of the ridge of the mandible shown in the previous figure and demonstrate the narrowness of the bony crest anteriorly.

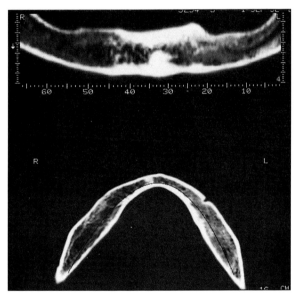

2.8 These CAT scans of the mandible shown in 2.2 demonstrate its thin cortex, lack of cancellous bone and labio-lingual thinning anteriorly.

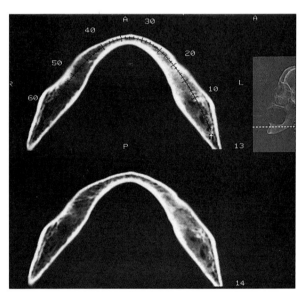

2.10 This slice of the mandible shown in 2.9 demonstrates that, even relatively close to the lower border, the jaw is still thin labio-lingually in the anterior region, which would present problems in implant insertion.

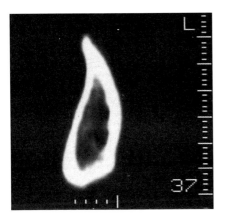

2.11 This traverse slice of the mandible shown in the previous figure demonstrates the narrow lip of bone on the crest of the jaw. If implants were to be inserted in this region this would need be to surgically reduced.

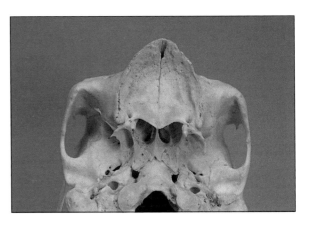

2.12 The maxilla undergoes severe resorption following tooth loss.

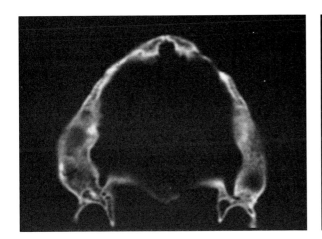

2.13 A CAT scan of the maxilla shown in 2.12 demonstrates the marked lack of bone near the ridge crest.

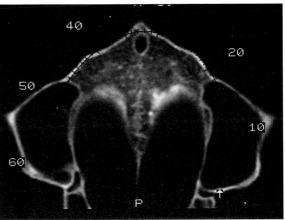

2.14 A scan taken at a more apical level shows that the maxillary sinuses involve much of the residual ridge and that there is little bone anteriorly.

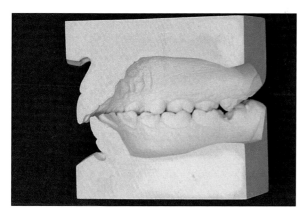

2.15 Sectioned casts of a dentate patient with a Type I incisor relationship.

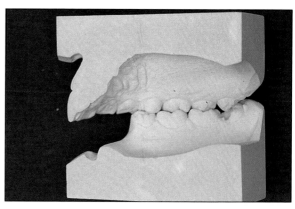

2.16 The cast in 2.15 trimmed to demonstrate the anticipated relationship of the lower edentulous ridge to the dentate maxilla, based on known patterns of alveolar resorption. The problems of restoring implants placed in the anterior mandible are evident.

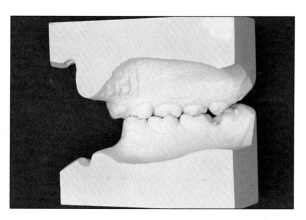

2.17 The anticipated relationship of the anterior mandible and maxilla following tooth loss. Comparison with 2.15 demonstrates the tissue deficit which it would be necessary to correct with prostheses.

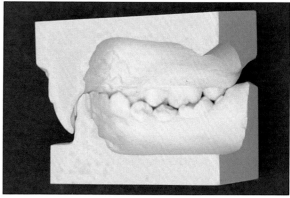

2.18 A Type II2 incisor relationship can present problems if it is to be reconstructed using prostheses following tooth loss.

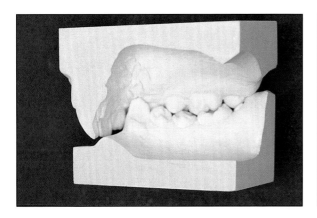

2.19 The difficulties of replacing this patient's anterior teeth with an implant-stabilised prosthesis are evident from these sectioned casts.

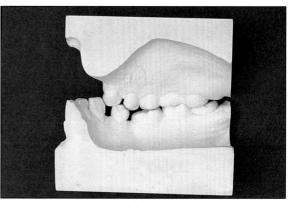

2.20 The replacement of this patient's anterior teeth with an implant-stabilised prosthesis will require a considerable amount of cantilevering as a result of the Class III apical base relationship and the alveolar resorption in the anterior maxilla.

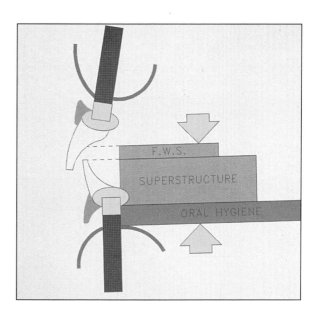

2.21 This diagram demonstrates the components of the vertical space which are required for an implant-stabilised fixed-bridge prosthesis.

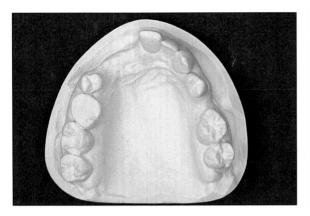

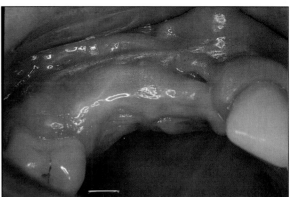

2.22–2.25 These figures illustrate a dental cast of a patient who had lost the upper right canine and incisor teeth in a road traffic accident. Whilst the cast and the clinical appearance suggest that treatment with an implant-stabilised prosthesis might be feasible, the CAT scans shown in 2.24 and 2.25 indicate that there is inadequate bone to place implants even at the level of the apices of the molar teeth.

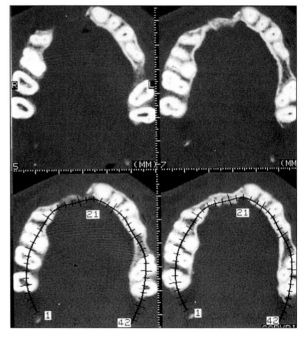

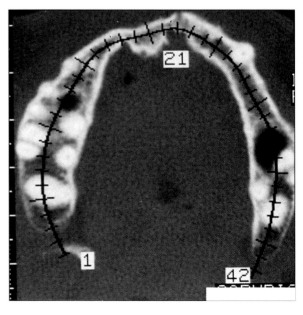

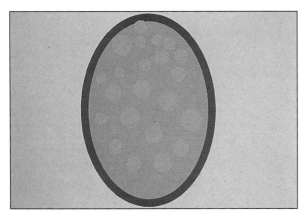

2.26 Where the jaw has a thin cortex surrounding sparse cancellous bone the prognosis for successful osseointegration is poor.

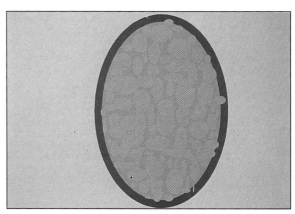

2.27 Despite a relatively thin cortex, bone with a dense inner core of cancellous material provides a better prognosis for successful implantation.

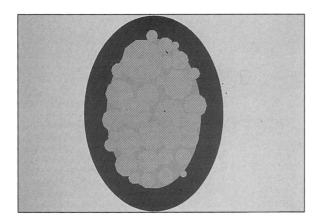

2.28 The combination of a dense cortex with diffuse cancellus bone can provide successful integration, particularly if the implant can transfix the bone so as to be inserted into both cortices.

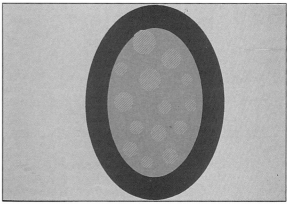

2.29 Where a thick dense cortex surrounds dense cancellous bone, surgical preparation is difficult and there is a considerable risk of thermal trauma to the bone. However, the prognosis for successful integration is good provided that these factors are taken into consideration.

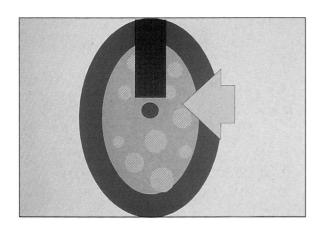

2.30 Where the mandibular canal is located centrally in the body of the mandible there may be inadequate space for the insertion of implants.

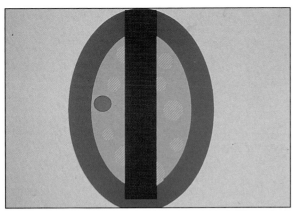

2.31 Lateral positioning of the mandibular canal can permit the use of longer implants. Such configurations are best confirmed using a tomogram.

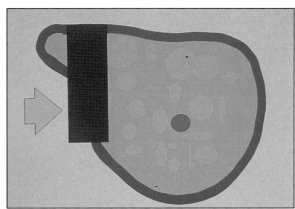

2.32 The body of the mandible often has a reduced thickness lingually and the placing of implants to avoid the mandibular canal can result in involvement with the floor of the mouth.

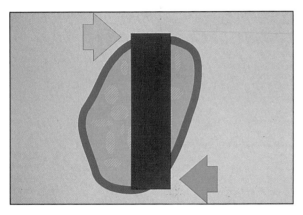

2.33 Although a lateral radiograph of the body of the mandible may suggest adequate room for implant insertion, the contours of the jaw may result in penetration of the cortices both superiorly and inferiorly. Penetration of the lower border usually heals by appositional bone growth. Failure to place the top of the implant level with the superior cortex can create problems with wound breakdown, or the top of the implant being above the level of the mucosal cuff following abutment placement.

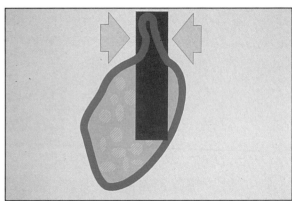

2.34 Where the ridge has a narrow crest, as shown in 2.11, this must be reduced before implants are inserted if they are to be seated within bone.

3. Selecting an Implant System

Introduction

Implants are devices inserted into the body below the skin or oral mucosal membrane, which they may penetrate, for the purpose of modifying form and function of the jaws or face, usually by mechanical means. Dental implants are those which are used in the oral cavity with the intention of improving the stability of a dental prosthesis. They have a history almost as old as that of dentistry itself. For most of this period they have been dominated by the belief that success was predominantly design-related, although more recently the importance of the material of construction was also recognised. The biological, as opposed to biomechanical, aspects of their applications were not, however, scientifically considered until recent decades. Allegorical reports on the success of treatment were common and whilst there were some considerable successes, predictability was poor, giving the technique an uncertain reputation.

Three principal types of device have been used: totally buried, subperiosteal and endosseous.

Now that endosseous dental implants can predictably provide a high degree of success, there is a large and growing number of systems on the market. All claim particular merits which may relate to performance, cost, ease of use or versatility. In some cases these claims are based on published research, in others their scientific basis is less evident. The largest amount of robust clinical data which are currently available relate to the Swedish O.I. Brånemark system. This partly reflects the period for which it has been available, but it should not be assumed that lack of data necessarily reflects lack of quality. It does, however, reduce the predictability, though not necessarily the success, of the outcome of treatment – a point which should be clear to operator and patient before the procedure starts.

In addition to an expanding range of implants, a market has appeared for the manufacture of specialised components where producers/developers are thought to be failing to meet a clinical need. These are often produced in a range

- **The totally buried** type of implant was typified by the ridge augmentation technique in which the height of a resorbed alveolar ridge was increased with an implant. Various ceramics were popular for this, as were a number of polymer-based materials such as 'Proplast', a carbon fibre/PTFE composite. There were often surgical problems in producing a significant increase in ridge height which was stable over an extended period and did not become infected. In addition there is no significant body of scientific evidence of the prosthetic benefits of the technique.

- **Subperiosteal** implants have principally been used in the atrophic mandible. They consist of a cast metal frame which fits the jaw bone and has projections into the oral cavity on which a prosthesis may be mounted. The frame is usually made from cobalt chromium alloy on a cast prepared from an impression

of the jaw bone. The technique can provide a very satisfactory result in the short term. However, over periods in excess of 15 years, failures tend to become more common. The implant–host interface is a fibrous one and oral epithelial down-growth eventually occurs around the implant. It is this which is believed to be the cause of the long-term failure of these devices.

- **Endosseous** dental implants have been manufactured as essentially blade, nail or screw-like devices inserted through the oral mucosa into the jaw bone. They have been produced in a wide range of shapes and materials and, until recently, had an uncertain prognosis. Recent work, particularly by P.-I. Brånemark and colleagues, has led to considerable developments in the field and the endosseous cylindrical design is now often thought of as being synonymous with a dental implant.

of designs for use with a variety of implant systems. Unfortunately the interchangeability of components between different manufacturers' ranges, and sometimes within them, is very restricted. As a result, clinicians tend to become familiar with one or two systems and may face problems when treating a patient who has an unfamiliar type of fixture.

Whilst it is possible to make detailed comparisons between implant systems the complexity of many ranges makes this difficult. The information also soon becomes dated as the field develops. Nevertheless, there are a number of generic characteristics of implants which are not specific to a particular manufacturer and which can be considered when choosing a system. These include its reported success, material of construction, design characteristics and the commercial support available.

Clinical success

The success of dental implantation is difficult to define; nevertheless, the criteria proposed by Albrektsson et al. (1986) are widely accepted and form a reproducible means of comparing systems. They have been used by a number of workers to follow the long-term success of endosseous dental implants, and their key features are summarised in **Table 3.1**.

When considering reported success for an implant system it is important to bear the following points in mind:

- Was the study carried out by the team which developed the system, or was the investigation an independent trial? Even with the greatest care the developers of a system tend to have more clinical success than independent workers.

- Were the patient groups comparable? The success of implant treatment is influenced by many variables. Unless these have been controlled they can affect the outcome of a study.

- Were the treatments similar in terms of type of superstructure and clinical situation in which they were employed?

- Was the data published in a peer-reviewed journal or contained solely in the manufacturer's own literature? Whilst manufacturers may pursue extremely high standards, independent work inevitably carries more weight.

Table 3.1. Criteria for success of dental implantation.

Clinical immobility of the fixture
Ability of the fixture to transmit masticatory loads without loss of integration
Absence of symptoms related to use of the implant
No damage to adjacent structures
Absence of progressive peri-implant radiolucency
Minimal progressive loss of crestal bone height

Implant material

The material from which a dental implant is manufactured can have a profound effect on the subsequent performance of the device. This relates not only to the nature of the interaction between the implant and the surrounding tissues, but also to the physical properties of the material, as these influence its behaviour under load. The biological response to materials is discussed in Chapter 1, and three broad groups, metals, ceramics and polymers, may be recognised.

Metals

Historically metals and their alloys have been the most widely used group of materials for implant construction, a situation which still exists. Currently commercially pure titanium (CPTi) is viewed as the best material from the viewpoint of tissue response. The reaction is nevertheless influenced by surface preparation and contamination, and the nature of the oxide layer on the surface of the metal. In addition, it is important to consider the design and use of the device, including patient factors, as these can markedly alter the performance of the implant.

Due to the desirable biological response which CPTi can elicit when suitably implanted in bone and the good long-term success of the Brånemark implant system, which uses this material, many other manufacturers now also employ this metal. The designs and construction of their implants are however different.

Unfortunately titanium is very sensitive to the inclusion of oxygen and is difficult to machine accurately. Its physical properties also make it less than ideal for fabricating small load-bearing dental components. As a result, some manufacturers have employed various titanium alloys, notably titanium/vanadium/aluminium, which have more suitable physical properties. There have been some suggestions based on histologic data that these elicit a response which is less favourable when implanted in bone, although long-term data are as yet restricted.

Stainless steel and cobalt/chromium/molybdenum alloys were at one time used for implant construction, but have largely been discarded as they do not readily integrate with bone and are prone to corrode. Other metals such as tantalum and zirconium have shown potential as load-bearing implantable materials but are not yet marketed as such.

Ceramics

The considerable chemical inertness of many ceramics and the similarities of one, hydroxyapatite, to the mineral of bone have made them attractive materials for implant production. They can be produced in a wide range of formulations, some of which readily become integrated when implanted in bone. Others are designed to be more reactive and are sometimes referred to as bioactive. Whilst this ill-defined characteristic may reflect a greater tendency to react chemically with the biological environment, it can also result in long-term degradation of the physical properties of the material as well as undesirable tissue changes.

Unfortunately the high moduli of elasticity of most ceramics, and their tendency to catastrophic failure in tension, create problems when using them for load transmission. In addition they cannot be easily formed into small precision components which dental systems often demand. This places constraints on the design of the implant. Only a very strong ceramic, such as microcrystalline alumina, can be used without reinforcement to make a dental implant. Other, weaker, ceramics such as hydroxyapatite, have to be used in combination with a metal, usually in the form of a coating. Whilst such coatings readily become integrated, the method of applying them can result in variations in their physical properties. Their method of attachment to the substrate is also largely mechanical and there have been occasional reports of delamination in service.

Other ceramics which are currently employed for implant construction include high purity microcrystalline alumina and single sapphire crystals.

Polymers

Whilst polymers have shown themselves to be very versatile in many novel engineering applications they have not, to date, proved successful for implant fabrication. This is due to the problems of obtaining integration, which is currently considered essential for the success of an endosseous implant. Their applications are therefore limited to the components of some implant systems where their physical properties are useful and the tissue responses which they invoke when implanted are appropriate. Examples of these applications are the elastomeric sealing 'O' ring on the abutment screw of a Brånemark implant, polymeric healing caps and the 'elastic' Intra-Mobile element of the IMZ implant system (**3.43, 3.44**).

Whilst the microporous PTFE membranes used for guided tissue regeneration are not dental implants in the traditional sense, they do represent another application of a polymer—being used where the influence of the implant on tissue behaviour is as essential to its application as that of an endosseous dental implant.

Design

The designs of dental implants demonstrate considerable diversity, some of which is considered in the section dealing with applications. A number of key features can be identified.

One- and two-stage designs

One-stage dental implants are intended to be inserted endosseously and to penetrate the oral mucosa from the time of insertion. This greatly simplifies the design of the device as the operator is presented from the start with a mechanical link which penetrates the mucosa. This has many similarities with an endodontically treated root, with or without an integral post depending on the design. As a result, a wide range of familiar techniques for producing a restoration is readily available.

The disadvantages of the technique are the need to penetrate the mucoperiosteum from the time of implant insertion. It has been argued that this will result in the application of external loads to the implant and allow epithelial down-growth around the fixture, both of which may prevent the formation of an osseointegrated interface. A further consideration is the increased risk of infection of the critical implant–host interface in its early stages. Unlike a two-stage system it is also impracticable to keep some implants in an unrestored state as 'sleepers' for possible use if another implant fails.

Once the dental arch is ready to be restored, a further problem can emerge as the location of the junction between the fixture and the super-structure is determined by the position of the top of the implant. Whilst posteriorly the junction may be positioned above the mucosal cuff, patients usually prefer the improved appearance of anterior margins which are placed below the mucosal cuffs. These must not be too deep, however, as this causes difficulties in producing a superstructure which fits well, due to the problems of accurately recording the position of a deeply placed implant. Unfortunately, accurate positioning of the top of a one-stage type of implant is complicated by the need to predict the mucosal contours once healing is completed.

Implants which are positioned and activated in two surgical stages are currently more widely used and embody a component which is totally buried at the time of first-stage surgery. Once this has become integrated it is exposed and finally a superstructure is added. The abutment which is added to the fixture is usually placed in two stages, the first of which involves using healing abutment to penetrate the mucosa. When the mucosal cuff is healed a definitive abutment is positioned. A superstructure is then placed on this, usually in the form of a fixed prosthesis or removable denture.

Such a design overcomes all the disadvantages of the single-stage system, but does introduce some new problems. The need to bury the implant makes its positioning more difficult, although in practice this can be overcome with a template. There can also be problems with bone growing over the top of the implant whilst it is buried. Once the abutment is placed, further problems can arise due to the need to use linkages which will prevent rotation and resist tensile moments. The abutment is nonetheless a versatile device which can provide considerable flexibility in superstructure design and placement.

Linkages

The method selected by the manufacturer to link the implant components may also be significant. Most provide resistance to rotation by means of lack of symmetry around the long axis of related components. This is often done with mating hexagonal surfaces on the opposing ends of two components. The resistance to separation by tension or torquing may be provided either with screws or by an adhesive.

Screws are inevitably more complex and thus result in a more expensive device. They require additional tools, are difficult to handle and are prone to wear and fracture if abused by the clinician or the patient. Once broken they may be difficult or sometimes impossible to retrieve. Screw linkages provide the significant advantage of ready retrievability. This makes it easy to replace worn components, to dismantle the system for checking and to alter the design of the superstructure if circumstances dictate.

Cemented joints are much simpler to design and use. They can also be used to compensate for deficiencies in the fit of mating components as in the CEKA Precidisk system, but are by definition not readily retrievable unless they can be forcefully broken. In addition they are less predictable as they depend on a bond which is usually predominantly mechanical, and have a less certain behaviour in the oral environment. When an adhesive is used to place an abutment there is also the potential for the material to be harmful to the gingival cuff either mechanically or chemically.

The simplicity, ease of use and space filling attributes of cemented joints make them valuable where their disadvantages are not critical.

Flexibility of design

The flexibility of design of a dental implant system is a crucial factor as it greatly extends the range of patients which may be treated and the types of device which can be placed on a fixture. The range of components available is a useful measure of flexibility, provided that this is based in a sound design.

Fixture sizes

The availability of a range of sizes of implant in terms of both length and diameter is important. In practice the range of diameters is limited by anatomical and design considerations. Most manufacturers make devices of about 4 mm in diameter, with narrower and broader devices in some ranges with diameters of the order of 3 and 5 mm. Broader implants are sometimes marketed as 'oversize', and are intended to be inserted where a narrower device has failed to be mechanically gripped by the bone at the time of insertion. This can arise as a result of surgical error or because the bone is relatively flexible.

Implant lengths will depend on location. In the maxilla it is often difficult to use longer implants, and thus devices as short as 7 mm may be chosen, although the success rate of these in the maxilla is markedly lower than devices about 10 mm long. In the lower jaw, implants are often placed to engage in both cortices and thus implants up to 20 mm are often needed.

Transmucosal abutments

The transmucosal abutment (TMA) is a crucial component in any two-stage implant system as it provides the essential link between fixture and superstructure. Of importance is the range of lengths of abutments and the availability of parallel-sided, tapering and angulated types, as well as of healing abutments.

A wide range of lengths will enable the clinician to handle different mucosal thicknesses and ensure that the space between the superstructure and the underlying mucosa has the optimum height. Abutments which are too short may make cleaning difficult, whilst those which are too long create problems in positioning the prosthesis and in restoring the implant. Shouldered abutments allow the use of superstructures in which the margin of the restoration is placed 'sub-gingivally'. This is essential for single crowns and prostheses placed anteriorly. It is helpful if the abutments have a range of shoulder heights as this facilitates placing the restoration margins just below the orifice of the mucosal cuff.

Healing abutments are made by some manufacturers and are intended for placement at the second stage of surgery whilst healing takes place. During this period there is often a change in the height of the gingival margin and the use of this type of abutment enables the correct length to be chosen once healing has occurred.

Temporary components

The construction of implant superstructures inevitably requires several clinical stages during which the patient will have to wear a temporary restoration. The availability of a range of disposable components to assist in making temporary appliances can considerably facilitate treatment, although it is not essential.

Prosthetic components

The link between the TMA or implant and the prosthesis is a crucial one, which is usually made via a manufactured component. This is designed to be incorporated into the superstructure and then joined to the remainder of the device with an adhesive or a screw. As superstructures are frequently made of a gold alloy it is usual to make the component of a similar material. This enables it to be soldered to the superstructure or cast on to. Superstructures for tapered abutments are often made of either porcelain or gold alloy, so that they can be incorporated into a porcelain crown or a metal-bonded ceramic restoration.

Most manufacturers provide at least one size of gold cylinder. However, components for ceramic restorations may be less readily available. A range of sizes will also increase the versatility of the system.

Commercial support

The availability of commercial support for the product by the manufacturer can be crucial. This includes a reliable system of quality control including batch numbers to enable faulty components to be rapidly identified and isolated. Such a system can also aid treatment by a different practitioner as particular components may be identified. The very long potential life of a dental implant will eventually result in many patients seeking care for restorations made on implants inserted many years before. The availability of accurate records will be essential if the dentist now treating the patient is to be able to identify the system and devices used.

When considering implant systems, the operator should also consider the resources of the manufacturer and whether he is in a position to provide effective support for the patient and his dentist for the lifetime of the fixtures. A period which may be the same as the patient's life expectancy, even in the young!

Support from one's professional colleagues is also important. All implant systems have their own characteristics and the availability of a colleague more experienced with a particular system can be helpful. This can also justify the joint purchase of specialised and rarely used instruments.

Costs

Whilst a detailed consideration of costs would be out of place in a book such as this, the reader should remember that they are not synonymous with price, and include the capital required to use the system, stock holding costs where there are delays in acquiring components, and maintenance costs where components need to be regularly replaced.

Terminology

The increasing use of dental implants has created its own terms. Some have been introduced by manufacturers, and are often specific to their product, others have been borrowed from different areas of dentistry or introduced specifically by clinicians and technicians. We do not propose to add to the vocabulary but include here the more commonly used terms in current use.

When carrying out implant treatment a suitable hole is prepared in the bone and a **fixture** inserted.

- A **fixture** may also be referred to as an **implant fixture** or an **implant**. Confusingly, the term **implant** may also be used to describe the fixture and all the components which may be mounted directly upon it to make up a complete unit.

To prevent bone growth over the fixture and into the hole in its centre it is covered with a **cover screw**. This is usually made of metal, but some manufacturers also make a similar polymeric device. Where a cemented linkage between components is used the cover screw may have a plain dowel rather than a screw thread.

Once the fixture has become integrated it is exposed in a second operation and an **abutment** placed on it. An abutment is a device which links the top of the fixture to the oral cavity and a wide range is available. These include:

- **Healing abutments** which are placed temporarily on the fixture whilst the soft tissues around them heal. These usually have a slightly greater diameter than the fixture.
- **Parallel abutments** which have parallel sides and have the superstructure mounted on top of them.
- **Tapered abutments** which enable the margin of the **superstructure** to be brought to or below the level of the mucosal cuff. These may or may not have a shoulder.
- **Angulated abutments** enable the orientation of the superstructure to be different to that of the fixture.

Because abutments penetrate the mucosa they are sometimes referred to as **trans-mucosal abutments** or **TMAs**.

The abutments are linked to the fixture with a cemented joint or an **abutment screw**.

Once the abutments have been mounted on the fixtures it is usual to place a **healing cap** on them.

- **Healing caps** are usually polymeric and are designed to protect the top of the abutment. Some are also shaped to hold a pack against the mucosal cuff in the period immediately after second-stage surgery. Healing caps may be held in place with friction or a screw fixing.

Impressions may be taken either of the top of the fixture or more commonly the abutment. To ensure accuracy this is done with **impression copings**.

Once the impression has been recorded a **replica abutment**, or **replica fixture**, is placed on the coping before the impression is poured. These are metal or polymeric devices supplied by the manufacturer to enable an accurate representation of the fixture or abutment to be incorporated in the cast.

- **Impression copings** are manufactured devices intended to be placed on the fixture or abutment and picked up in the impression. They may be held in place by friction, an integral screw or a separate screw.

A superstructure is then produced and mounted on the abutment(s). A wide range of prostheses may be placed on the implants, and these are either fixed or removable (patient removable).

A popular method of linking the superstructure to an abutment is with a **gold cylinder** or **coping**, which may be manufactured or prepared by casting a plastic pattern.

Fixed superstructures are analogous to fixed bridges and are often referred to as **implant-stabilised fixed prostheses** to avoid confusion with conventional bridges and those supported by teeth and implants.

- The gold cylinder is manufactured to be a precision fit on the abutment, and may include anti-rotation features in its design. It is usually incorporated into the superstructure by casting the framework on to it. Frameworks are usually made of gold alloy, although other materials including titanium are sometimes used. The cylinder then acts as the fixing point for the superstructure and is usually held in place with a **gold cylinder screw**.

Where single crowns are placed on implants manufacturers usually provide a **ceramic core**, **metal core** or **castable plastic pattern** to act as a foundation for the crown.

The terminology for extra-oral implants is similar to those for intra-oral use.

Illustrations

The illustrations in this section show a number of implant systems. These are almost entirely designs which are presently available from manufacturers. They have been used to demonstrate the principles described above and the inclusion of a particular system, or in some cases the demonstration of a failed component, is not intended to reflect any beneficial or adverse characteristics of that system.

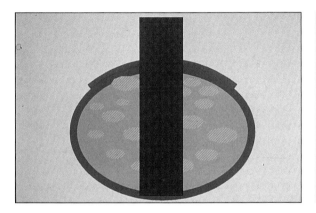

3.1 Fixtures which penetrate the mucosa from the time of insertion require only a single surgical procedure. There may be problems associated with their immediate penetration of their mucosa.

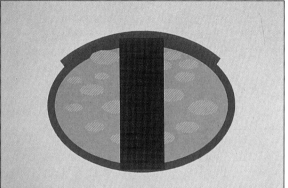

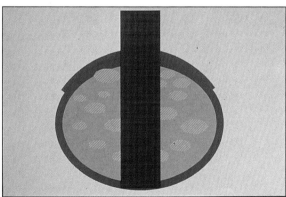

3.2, 3.3 Fixtures which are initially buried and later have an abutment placed in a second surgical procedure permit undisturbed healing of the tissues around the implant.

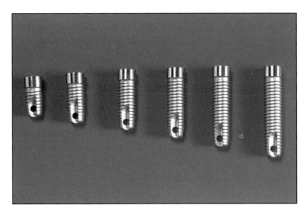

3.4 Most manufacturers provide a range of implant lengths and diameters. Screw-shaped devices can provide good initial fixation. [S]

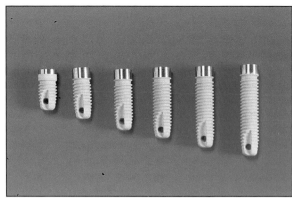

3.5 This manufacturer also provides a range of hydroxyapatite-coated threaded implants. [S]

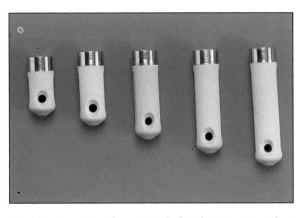

3.6 Hydroxyapatite-coated implants are also available in a non-threaded form. [S]

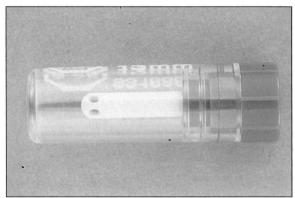

3.7 Most manufacturers supply their fixtures in sealed sterile containers, such as this Calcitek-coated implant.

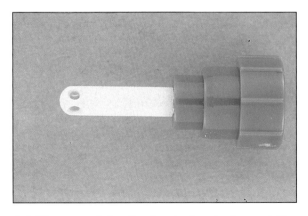

3.8 The mount for the implant acts to seal the container and is a simple carrier for positioning the implant fixture in the bony canal.

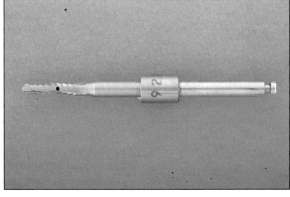

3.9 An internally irrigated drill used in the preparation of a canal to accept a Calcitek implant.

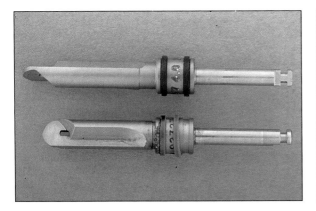

3.10 A spade drill used to gouge bone.

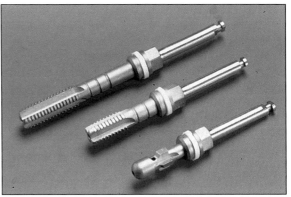

3.11 Thread-forming or cutting drill bits are used with threaded implants. [S]

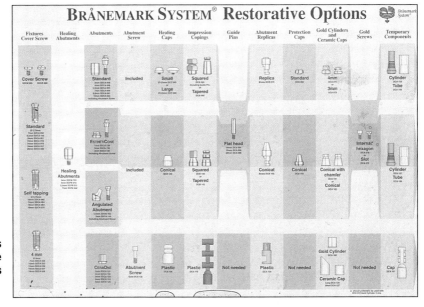

3.12 Several manufacturers provide a comprehensive range of components which increases the flexibility of the system.

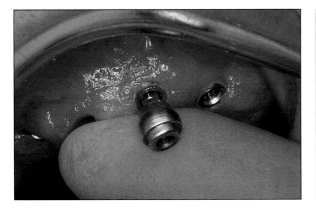

3.13, 3.14 Abutments may be joined to fixtures using a spigot, which may have an irregular profile to prevent rotation. These are cemented in place.

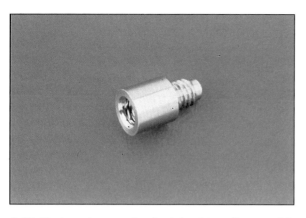

3.15 Abutments may also be joined to a fixture with an integral screw. [S]

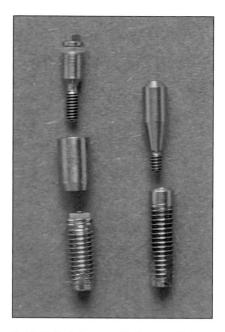

3.16 Nobelpharma (Brånemark) and Astra fixtures with abutments with separate and integral screws.

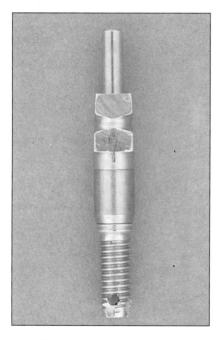

3.17 Nobelpharma fixture with TMA and coping.

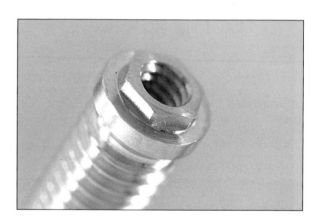

3.18 The Brånemark fixture incorporates an hexagonal head to prevent rotation. The threaded internal hole for mounting the abutment can be seen.

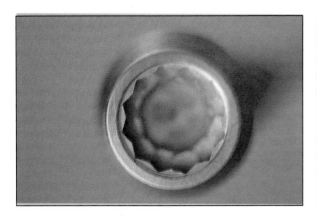

3.19 The surface of an angulated abutment for use with the fixture shown in 3.18. The internal machining prevents rotation and provides for a range of positions.

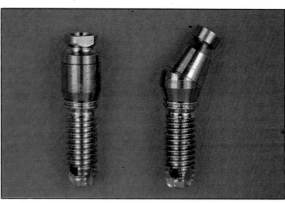

3.20 The Brånemark angulated abutment with gold cylinder.

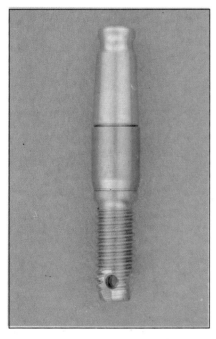

3.21 Brånemark fixture with TMA and round coping.

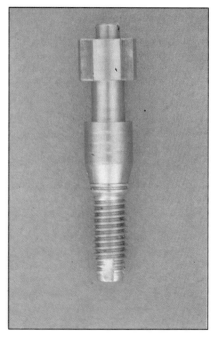

3.22 Brånemark fixture with direct coping.

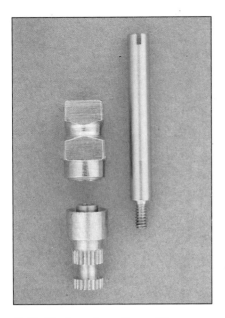

3.23 Abutment replica with screw and coping.

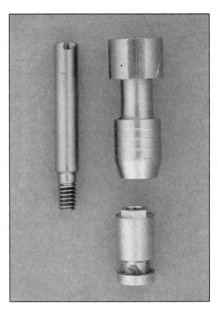

3.24 Fixture replica with direct coping and screw.

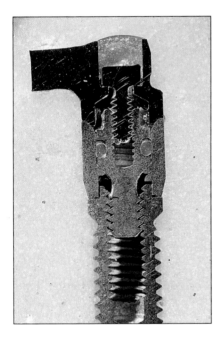

3.25 Ground longitudinal section of a Brånemark implant fixture with abutment and gold cylinder incorporating part of an overdenture bar. This demonstrates the various components and the complexity of the assembled device.

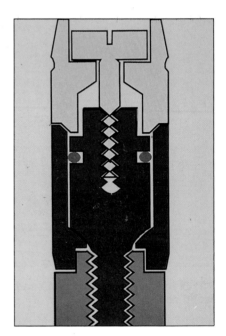

3.26 This diagram of an assembled implant shows the fixture (grey), the abutment (red), and abutment screw (purple), surmounted by the gold cylinder and gold cylinder screw (yellow). The elastomeric sealing ring (orange) is incorporated by some manufacturers to prevent the ingress of fluid.

3.27 The internal mating of the fixture with the Omniloc abutment indicates a variety of choices of precise positions for the abutment when the two are secured with an abutment screw. [C].

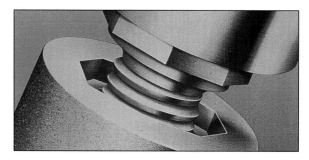

3.28 Diagrams indicating the seating of the abutment into the Calcitek fixture. Principle of seating (left); using tool to seat abutment (right) [C].

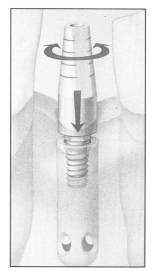
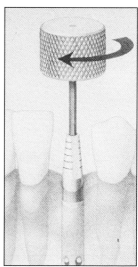

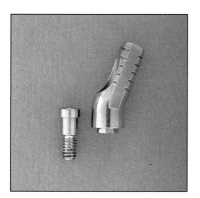
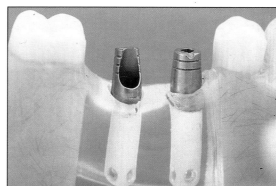

3.29 Pre-angled abutment (upper left); straight and angled abutment *in situ* (upper right); molar crown cemented and pre-molar screwed in place (lower left); straight and pre-angled Omniloc abutments (lower right).

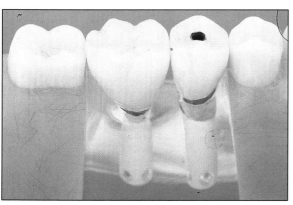
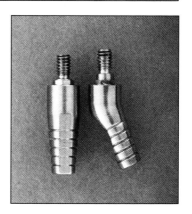

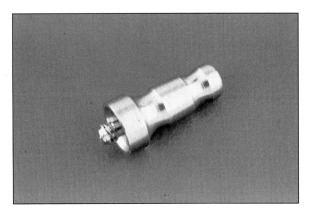

3.30 Impression copings may be joined to the abutments with an integral screw. [S]

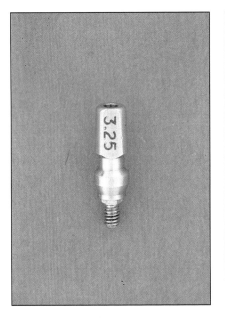
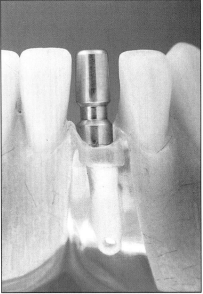

3.31 An impression post (coping) used directly with the fixture. [C]

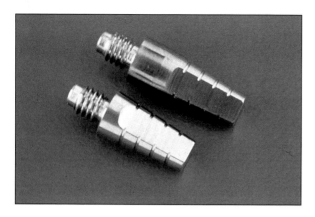

3.32 Shoulderless abutments for use with cemented restorations are provided by some manufacturers. [S]

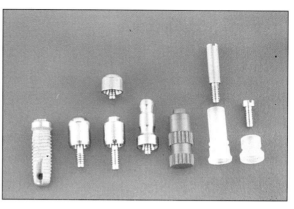

3.33 This manufacturer provides a range of components for restoring the fixture on the left of the picture. To the right are two abutments, an impression coping, a replica abutment for laboratory use (blue) and castable plastic patterns. [S]

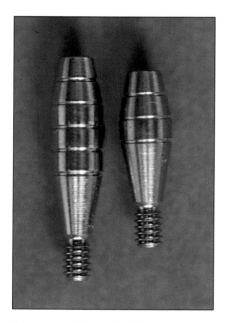

3.34 The Astra implant system uses an extended type of healing cap.

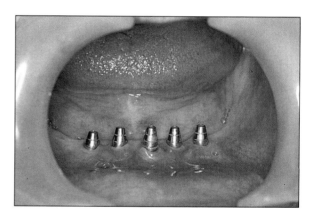

3.35 Astra healing caps in use.

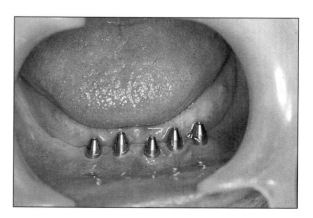

3.36 Once the mucosal cuff has healed after second-stage surgery the healing caps are replaced with abutments, -20 degrees tapered pattern.

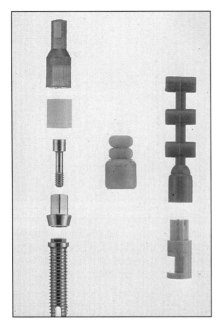

3.37 Components used by the Brånemark system for a single tooth restoration. On the left are the fixture, shouldered abutment and abutment screw, ceramic sleeve and castable plastic pattern. A healing cap, polymeric replica abutment and impression coping are on the right. [N]

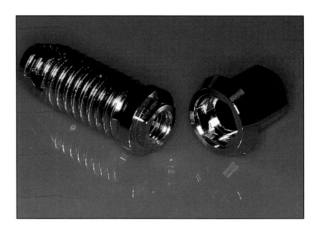

3.38 A Nobelpharma fixture and shouldered abutment demonstrating the hexagonal coupling to prevent rotation. [N]

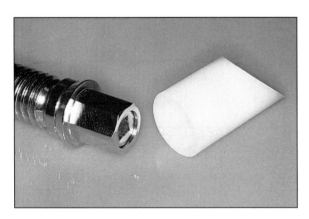

3.39 A ceramic sleeve for use with this shouldered abutment. The sleeve forms the core of a porcelain crown and the hexagonal abutment resists its rotation. [N]

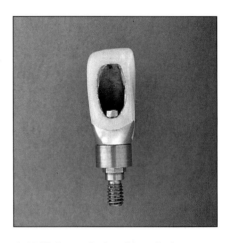

3.40 Universal shouldered abutment and screw (prosthesis screwed in position).

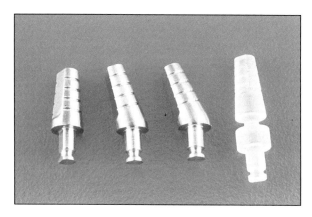

3.41 Some manufacturers provide a range of angulated abutments. Also seen here is a plastic pattern for producing a cast abutment. [S]

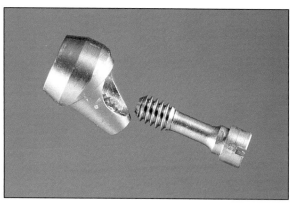

3.42 An angulated screw-retained, abutment for use with the Brånemark implant system.

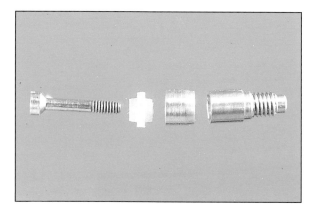

3.43, 3.44 One manufacturer incorporates a polymeric component in the abutment system to act as a shock absorber. The plastic component is inserted between the abutment and the fixture as shown in 3.43.

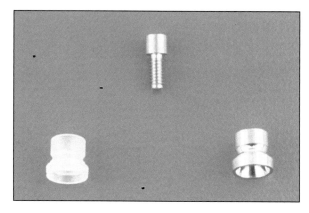

3.45 Manufactured gold cylinders may be incorporated into cast superstructures and are usually screw-retained. Some manufacturers also provide plastic patterns for cylinder production. [S]

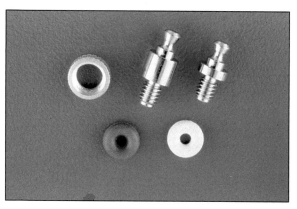

3.46 Abutments used for denture stabilisation with polymeric O rings which are inserted into the fitting surface of the denture. [S]

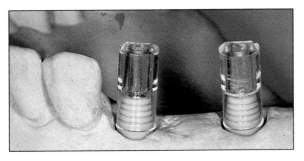 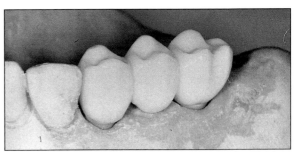

3.47, 3.48 Components for the construction of temporary prostheses (3.48, right) facilitate the restoration of implants whilst permanent appliances are being made. [N]

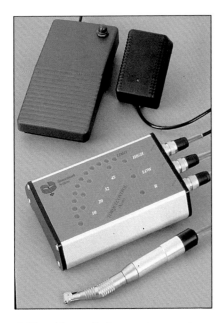

3.49 All manufacturers provide a range of tools for use with their implant systems. These are usually manufacturer-specific. [S]

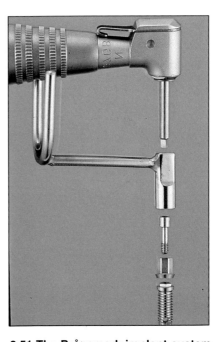

3.50 The Brånemark system employs an electronically controlled mechanical driver for tightening the various screws to the correct torque. [N]

3.51 The Brånemark implant system incorporates a counter torque device which is placed over the abutment to prevent twisting of the fixture whilst the abutment screw is tightened. (See also 7.86)

4. Patient Assessment

Introduction

The decision to provide implant treatment should be made upon firm evidence that rehabilitation will confer long-term benefit to the patient and will produce a superior result to other alternative procedures of replacing a defective or totally deficient dentition with conventional bridges or dentures (**4.1–4.5**). This view is in contrast to the wishes of some patients who demand only the apparent advantages of fixed tooth replacement, or of dentists whose appreciation has been limited to a consideration that sufficient space exists for positioning an implant in jaw bone. An appropriate history and dental examination will reveal systemic and local factors highly influential in reaching a prognosis for a treatment proposal.

It is especially important to recognise that successful rehabilitation with an implant-stabilised prosthesis should be matched with the same long-term prognosis for the remainder of the dentition. Likewise treatment of one jaw with osseo-integration techniques should not create future difficulties in the opposing jaw of an edentulous patient.

Relevant medical and dental history

> **Essential information**
> - What is the patient's complaint?
> - Why has the patient requested implant treatment?
> - Has the patient experienced successful routine prosthetic/restorative treatment?
> - Is the patient aware of the requirements for implant treatment and long-term success?

Information should be sought upon the attitude, occupation and general health of the patient. Two extremes in patient awareness should be guarded against. Those who eagerly anticipate that replacement will restore completely all oral functions and create the youthful appearance of natural teeth are unlikely to be easily satisfied with an artificial substitute. In contrast, those who have consistently neglected their dentition, having low standards of oral hygiene, will usually have insufficient interest to maintain their oral health and prostheses in good order (**4.6**). This will have potentially adverse effects upon tissue integration of the dental implant. This group is also not likely to wish to spend the time on sophisticated treatment or merit its costs. A further problem arises with those patients who claim to have received unsatisfactory prosthetic treatment resulting in loose or painful dentures or have experienced difficulty in controlling or tolerating them. Careful questioning, accompanying an examination of the mouth and denture, may confirm if the complaint is justified and indicate whether or not an alternative, satisfactory solution may be reached by simple routine denture treatment carried out to a high standard (**4.7**).

Some occupations contraindicate the use of dental implants, e.g. wrestlers and boxers where the risk of failure of intricate components is too high. Whereas those facing the public in demanding situations, e.g. teachers, wind instrumentalists and health-care professionals, may overcome the problems of the unwanted display of metal clasps or the embarrassment of wearing loose removable dentures by having a secure implant-stabilised prosthesis.

A history of retching, unassociated with a phobia concerning dental treatment, should be carefully assessed. Such problems may first appear when the patient loses a significant number of teeth and finds the wearing of dentures intolerable. The examination should confirm the trigger sites within the oral cavity and a decision must be made whether or not the patient is likely to tolerate the prosthodontic treatment necessary to provide even a small implant restoration sited anteriorly in the jaws (**4.8, 4.9**).

The general health status of the individual must also be properly considered. Implants are not recommended for the elderly, infirm person who is unable to undergo prolonged surgical treatment and subsequently to maintain high standards of oral health, or for those suffering psychiatric disorders (e.g. depression), or having drug or alcohol dependence where cooperation may fluctuate (**4.10, 4.11**). Likewise, patients compromised by elective surgery and infection, for example those with heart failure, mitral stenosis, uncontrolled diabetes, blood dyscrasias etc., should be counselled to avoid this type of treatment. Patients for whom implant integration is less certain, e.g. those having had recent irradiation of the jaws, would also be considered unsuitable. Conversely, careful thought should be given to the possible stabilisation of dentures or their replacement by a fixed prosthesis using implants for some patients exhibiting adverse neuromuscular control (e.g. cerebral palsy) where operative techniques are manageable and suitable, and where high standards of home care can provide effective levels of oral hygiene and maintenance. However, those patients whose manual dexterity is sufficiently limited so as to restrict severely their capacity to brush their teeth or dentures, e.g. those with arthritis of the hands, should be advised against seeking this form of treatment (**4.12**).

Medical history contraindicating treatment
- Infirm elderly
- Medical/surgical risk e.g: Uncontrolled diabetic
  Immuno-compromised
  Blood dyscrasia
  Impaired cardiovascular function
- Drug/alcohol dependence
- Psychiatric disorder e.g: Paranoia
  Dysmorphophobia
- Recent irridiation of oral, facial tissues
- Smoking (?heavy use)

Important features of extra-oral examination

A number of important extra-oral findings must be considered if implant treatment is to be feasible and the outcome satisfactory. It is essential that the operator has sufficient easy access to the oral cavity (**4.13**). The gape may be limited by previous trauma to the jaws or from pathological change (in cases of scleroderma, for example). The morphology of the lips with and without the presence of dentures in the mouth will indicate if a flange, and hence a removable prosthesis, is essential to provide an acceptable contour in order to mask the result of alveolar resorption (**4.14**). The function of the lips should also be observed when the patient smiles and speaks. If there is display of the alveolar process and the gingival tissue of the jaws, this will make the design of the prosthesis more difficult (**4.15**). It will not be acceptable for the patient to display titanium abutments. The artificial tooth crowns may subsequently appear abnormally long or incorrectly angulated, especially in comparison with adjacent natural teeth. Where a flange is required to restore the lip support and maintain the preferred arch shape, there may be display of the border together with the space required for access below the fixed prosthesis and to the mucosal cuffs. As a result, a removable implant-stabilised overdenture may be more appropriate than a fixed prosthesis for restoring an edentulous jaw.

Abnormalities of the lips arising from previous surgical intervention may make the access to the edentulous jaw sites difficult and result in distortion of the space available for the prosthesis. Such examples may be found in the repair of congenital clefts of the lip and palate and in the use of nasolabial flaps in the treatment of resection of the mandible.

Obvious disproportion and malalignment of the jaws (e.g. in skeletal class II or III patterns and associated with similar malocclusions) may hinder the design of an appropriate prosthesis (**4.16**). Lack of space for components within the mouth (**4.17**) and conflict between the positions of the fixtures and the required location of the artificial teeth in the arch should be considered in assessing the findings of the intra-oral examination (**4.18**).

Intra-oral examination – the partially edentulous patient

General considerations

When undertaking an examination of a partially edentulous individual two important questions should be borne in mind: (i) does the space in the dental arch need to be restored? (ii) does the patient exhibit a high standard of restorative care and have a stable periodontal status? (**4.19, 4.20**). If there are affirmative answers to both questions then an implant-stabilised partial prosthesis may have significant advantages over a conventional bridge which requires abutment tooth preparation and a removable partial denture which is likely to require greater tooth and soft-tissue coverage (**4.21**). Assessment should also predict that there is the likelihood of creating a pleasing appearance and producing stable posterior occlusal support.

Examination of the site of tooth loss may clearly indicate the advantage of implant treatment over alternative solutions. Loss of a single maxillary incisor tooth without the complications of space closure or excessive vertical overlap in the segment of the arch may allow a single tooth implant prosthesis to be sited. This is an especially attractive solution when the abutment teeth are unrestored. The alternative solution of using a resin-bonded bridge is more appropriate for youthful patients. Minimal tooth preparation is required and the bond may survive for a limited period (e.g. 4 years) until maturity is reached and there is less risk of accidental damage (**4.4**). Similarly, extensive tooth loss of all incisor and canine teeth may create a technically difficult solution requiring multiple clasping and compromised support for a partial denture or extensive crown preparation for a bridge, whereas a localised fixed partial prosthesis supported by implants may provide an ideal result.

Extensive distal extension removable prostheses are also difficult to manage, especially where an incisor tooth forms an unsuitable abutment for clasping and support (**4.22**). The option of implant treatment should be considered. However, multiple sites of tooth loss in the dental arch requiring replacement, including distal extensions, are usually more satisfactorily managed with a removable partial denture (**4.5**).

The motivation of the patient in maintaining good oral health, the periodontal status and the standard of restorative care, all of which reflect in the long-term survival of the dentition should be judged by the accepted approaches of restorative evaluation. Whilst neglected mouths, multiple poorly executed restorations of the teeth and advanced chronic periodontal disease, together with evidence of plaque-coated dentures, may clearly contraindicate the use of such sophisticated treatment, more difficult judgements arise with other situations (**4.19, 4.20**). The potential failure of an endodontically treated tooth with a split root, or loss of a key bridge abutment in an otherwise carefully restored dentition, may compromise an otherwise straightforward decision for implant treatment in another quadrant of the mouth. Hence, not only should the local span appropriate for restoration be examined but a judgement is required of those teeth considered to be vulnerable so that the results of examination may also predict where implant treatment may be unsuitable. One such example would be the loss of molar teeth adjacent to an extensive maxillary antrum where only a subsequent bone grafting procedure would allow their replacement by implant treatment.

Examination of the local site

Important local features

- Is the residual dentition healthy?
- Is there adequated gape for instrumentation?
- Does sufficient inter-tooth space allow positioning of fixture(s), abutment(s) and prosthesis?
- Does inter-arch space permit restoration?
- Is the occlusion stable, without evidence of excessive tooth surface loss?
- Is there over-eruption of opponent teeth?
- How many sites require restoration?
- Are the gingivae evident (e.g: 'high lip line')?
- Will the prosthesis replace coronal or coronal and alveolar tissue?

Initial inspection should confirm adequate access to the edentulous area of the jaw. The gape, especially between over-erupted teeth, may preclude the use of the correct fixture length, the fixture mount connector and handpiece head (**4.23**). A distance of 4 cm or more may be required to manipulate the handpiece and any less space may cause the operator to misalign the fixture, resulting in a poor position relative to the prosthetic tooth crown, or risking compromise of the adjacent tooth root. Even short screwdrivers for subsequent component linkage require a minimum of 2 cm above the prosthetic unit (e.g. in securing a transfer coping or abutment) (**4.24**).

The minimum distance between adjacent teeth should be adequate to enclose the fixture in a sufficient volume of bone without compromising the periodontal membranes (**4.25**). In the case of a 4 mm diameter implant, this span will be 6 mm. This will provide a minimum of 1 mm between the side of the implant and the adjacent periodontal membrane or another implant. In such a situation there is little tolerance for error in positioning the implant. However, close observation of the teeth may indicate tilting, with the resultant span having less distance between the roots (**4.26, 4.27**). (Special instruments are required for both surgical and prosthetic treatment of small spaces in the dental arch.) When replacing several teeth, one implant may support two artificial crowns, provided a minimum of two implant fixtures are used (**4.28**). Palpation and inspection of the residual ridge crest will indicate if the superior surface is adequately broad or if the buccal or lingual face is concave, so risking exposure of part of the fixture. Narrowing of the crest may dictate surgical reduction of the alveolus with the consequent reduction in fixture length and increase in dimension of the prosthesis. This, in turn, will affect the loading of the implant and alter the appearance of the prosthesis by requiring a longer crown or the supplementation with a flange in the prosthesis. Appraisal of the precise width may be accomplished by radiography and by ridge mapping with callipers to measure the thickness of bone directly (**4.29–4.31**).

The covering mucosa should be assessed for quality and mobility. Thick fibrous mucosa is likely to require the use of a long abutment and create a deep mucosal crevice. Unfavourable pathogens may colonise the crevice if the periodontal tissues of the residual dentition are unhealthy. Also, in the presence of a mobile cuff, the mucosa is likely to require a longer healing period after abutment connection.

Inspection of the level of the ridge mucosa, resulting from resorption, compared to the adjacent gingivae of the teeth bounding the edentulous span, will indicate whether or not the prosthesis may be constructed with crowns located on aesthetically designed abutments (e.g. Brånemark CeraOne System) or made with a flange to replace the missing alveolar tissue. Conventional parallel-sided abutments may be positioned with their superior surfaces at or above the level of the mucosa. Whereas tapered abutments (with or without a shoulder) can be used to place the junction with the prosthesis 'subgingivally' so that the margin of the crown or fixed prosthesis is within the mucosal cuff(s) without evidence of the titanium abutments. Confirmation of the decision may frequently require a set-up of an artificial tooth to be inspected at a trial insertion (**4.32, 4.33**; see Chapter 7).

Finally a comparison is required between the position of the adjacent natural tooth crown and the ridge to determine the likely position of the artificial crown and the possible cantilevering that may be expected away from the implant fixture. Also, divergence between the possible long axis of an implant fixture and the artificial tooth crown should be estimated so that consequences in the design of the prosthesis can be anticipated. Typical examples of this planning are consideration of the requirement for ridge lapping of the crown when the alveolus demands a palatal position for the implant, or the need to use an angulated abutment if the implant cannot be placed vertically in the alveolus beneath the prosthesis but is required to be inclined labially by the limitation of the jaw shape (see Chapter 7).

Examination of the occlusion

The usual routine appraisal of the dentate occlusion should be made (**4.34**). Evidence of a normal freeway space, a symmetrical undeviated path of jaw closure and the absence of obvious tooth surface facets of wear, associated with bruxism, should be recorded. Close relation between the retruded and intercuspal tooth contact positions without evidence of deflective premature contacts should be achieved. The area of natural tooth contact should be observed to indicate if the natural teeth or the prosthesis will provide the prime source of occlusal stability. In the case of single tooth replacement, it is important to assess if the planned artificial tooth crown could be subjected to sole eccentric tooth contact, e.g. create canine guidance because of the requirement for a deep overbite with a crown of suitable length (**4.35**). Where the occlusal plane is disturbed by over-eruption of unopposed teeth, articulated models are usually needed to supplement clinical evidence to confirm that sufficient space exists for the prosthesis and the abutments. A minimum of 6 mm for standard Brånemark abutments and 7.5 mm for angulated abutments is needed in the vertical plane. Treatment to avoid eccentric occlusal interferences may be required, for example by minimal enamel grinding or by reduction and crowning opposing teeth.

Intra-oral examination — the edentulous patient

Examining the edentulous jaw

Inspection of the jaw ridge produces an immediate impression of the possible volume of available bone. Not infrequently, those complaining of the difficulty of wearing loose and painful dentures lack a good well-rounded ridge, and palpation emphasises a narrow shallow form to the underlying bony ridge in the maxillae. However, palpation both across the anterior mandible and from the oral mucosa to the skin surfaces may indicate that the lack of alveolar bone is not necessarily associated with a deficit in the body of the jaw (**4.36, 4.37**). Evidence of a sharp ridge crest may indicate the potential to reduce it by alveolar surgery and leave sufficient bone to accept fixtures of 7 mm or more in length (**4.42**). Palpation of the maxillae may indicate the presence of buccal and labial concavities with consequent limitation of the jaw in the depth of the sulcus. Also the ridge may be found to consist of substantial amounts of displaceable fibrous tissue covering insufficient bone or creating a potentially deep cuff around the abutment secured upon a fixture.

Observation of the relation of the ridge with the opposing edentulous jaw or dentate arch is important. Using the existing complete dentures it is possible to determine the likely arch relation to the underlying jaw and so assess the potential cantilevering of the dental arch from the estimated position of implants in the jaw (**4.40, 4.41**). This is particularly important where an edentulous jaw opposes a complete natural arch of teeth and there is no opportunity to revise the arrangement of the artificial teeth in the intended prosthesis. More detailed planning can be achieved with articulated study casts. It is also important to consider the occlusal relation where a dentate arch opposes an edentulous jaw. The length of the occlusal table of the prosthesis reflects the length of the opposing arch as well as the location of potential implants. For example, it may be possible to oppose the natural dentition only with an implant-stabilised removable overdenture if the implant fixtures are restricted to the anterior mandible (**4.38, 4.39**). Otherwise, some natural teeth may require to be unopposed when a fixed cantilevered prosthesis is constructed with the necessarily shortened dental arch. Abnormalities in the position of individual natural teeth or of the inclination of the entire occlusal plane must be identified (e.g. over-eruption of several molar teeth) so that the effect of lack of space for the opposing prosthesis or the creation of eccentric tooth interferences, which in turn may create unfavourable stresses on the bone-implant interface, can be considered.

Careful examination of the existing complete dentures will indicate shortcomings in their design affecting the appearance, occlusion or support and stability of the dentures. Frequently, one denture is judged by the patient to be satisfactory and the request is for a solution to the problem of wearing the other. However, it is important not only to consider what changes, if any, are appropriate but also to consider the possible effect of providing a very stable fixed prosthesis in one jaw upon the hitherto satisfactory removable prosthesis in the other jaw. It is important to assess first if complete border seal is achievable, especially if the support tissues are atrophied and, secondly, if adequate stability of this denture is likely. (Where totally inadequate dentures exist, it is usually necessary to construct a replacement set as part of treatment.)

Radiographic assessment

Radiographs for assessment/monitoring

- Intra-oral dental (parallel and long-cone technique)
  Assessing inter-radicular space, bone quality
  Monitoring component fit, implant status
- Pan-oral
  Assessing general dental status, available bone height, location of vital structures
  Identifying implant location
  Monitoring prosthetic outcome
- CT scan—jaw, skull (reformatted image)
  Assessing precise volume of available bone and relation of vital structures in sequential image slices
- Tomogram—jaw (e.g: Scanora)
  Assessing in cross-section precise volume of available bone at selected sites in jaw, and relation of vital structures

Appropriate radiographs are essential to complement the evidence from the clinical examination in order to confirm the dental status, to determine the available volume and quality of bone in edentulous sites of the jaws, and to plan the treatment of the patient (**4.43**).

Routinely used radiographs should be recorded first. A standard dental periapical film recorded in the plane of a proposed implant will indicate, for example, the quality of the bone and the space available between adjacent teeth. Likewise, a standard orthopantomograph (OPG) will provide evidence of retained roots or other pathology in edentulous areas (**4.44, 4.45**), and the potential height (although magnified) to the jaws, especially

above the inferior dental canal along its course to the mental foramen and, in the upper jaw, below the maxillary antrum and beside the incisive fossa (**4.46**). The incorporation of a metal marker with a known length within the field (e.g. in a template) will allow closer estimation of the height of the jaw. Not infrequently, potentially well-shaped edentulous maxillary jaw ridges may be shown to be extensively occupied by the antrum or covered by a thick layer of fibrous tissue.

It is also essential to be aware of the thickness (width) of available bone (**4.47, 4.48**). This may be judged from a lateral skull radiograph when the cross-sectional form of the centre of the edentulous jaws may be determined. A variety of qualities and shapes are to be observed. Apart from knowledge of the depth and width of the jaw, together with evidence of the definition of the cortical plate and density of the trabecular bone within, this film may reveal unexpected narrowing and concavities which may adversely affect the placement of fixtures in sites close to the mid-line. The volume and quality of available bone is critical to the success of treatment, and characteristics of the quantity and quality of the available bone have been classified by Lekholm and Zarb. From the accompanying diagram it will be seen that registration in the highest number category indicates the poorest prognosis for the outcome of osseointegration and the response of the implant fixture to loading (**4.49**). As the patterns of resorption of the jaw are so variable, Cawood and Howell have increased the number of categories of shape. This is of significance in judging the need for grafting to augment the jaw and so permit the placement of implants (**4.50**).

Where the jaw form appears regular, if good quality and quantity of bone exist in the mid-line, it is likely that adjacent areas as far as the premolar zones will also provide suitable housing for the fixtures.

However, it is not uncommon for the clinician to be uncertain whether or not sufficient volume of bone exists at specific sites in the jaw. It is then appropriate to use sophisticated apparatus to secure reliable measurements of the available bone in which to place the implants and, in particular, to avoid damage to vital structures. The computerised tomograph (CT scan) and the tomograph (e.g. Scanora system; **4.31**) produce such detail. Specifically designed computer software for the CT scan enables a series of images to be generated both in the axial plane, producing horizontal slices through the jaws, and as a series of cross-sectional cuts made at right angles to the midplane of the jaw. By consulting the scale pictured in the radiographs and graduated to show millimetre widths, it is possible to determine the depth and width of the jaw at any of 32 sites. Information of similar quality is available in a more familiar form using the Scanora system. Prior to radiography, the sites selected for implantation are marked on a study model and a clear acrylic resin template is prepared carrying 1 mm metal markers above these sites (**4.30**).

The template is inserted into the mouth and a 'scout' orthopantomogram is recorded. From this information cross-sectional tomograms are then recorded at the sites of the markers. The interpretation of available bone is achieved using a rule supplied by the manufacturer and graduated to allow for the known magnification of the image. With either method it is possible to have reliable estimates from which to select an appropriate length and diameter of implant and to envisage how the morphology of the jaw may impact on the location and angulation of each implant.

In reaching a conclusion upon the volume of available bone, the operator may arrive at one of a number of decisions.

- Sufficient bone exists to encompass a fixture of appropriate dimension and that an appropriate number of fixtures can be placed to endorse the proposed treatment plan, e.g. five fixtures, 13 mm length, 3.75 mm diameter to support a fixed prosthesis in the anterior mandible.
- Insufficient width of bone exists to encompass a 3.75 mm diameter fixture, demanding the use of a guided tissue regeneration technique to provide enough bone to enclose the fixture. A thinner diameter fixture may be an appropriate alternative.
- Insufficient volume of bone requires the use of a bone graft to augment the jaw or the maxillary antrum to permit the use of both the residual jaw and the graft.
- Sufficient bone may exist to allow the fixture to be placed without damaging the adjacent periodontal membranes of the teeth, i.e. 6 mm to accommodate a 3.75 mm diameter fixture. However, the position of the fixture may conflict with the ideal design of the prosthesis. For example, considerable cantilevering is necessary to place the crown in the expected contour of the arch.
- Fixtures cannot be placed in some intended sites so that the design of the prosthesis must be changed.

Radiographic interpretation of the quality of the bone is less easily achieved. Examination of the lateral skull X-ray of the anterior mandible may indicate well-defined superior and inferior cortical surfaces with an almost radiolucent interior to the mid-line of the symphysis. A fixture secured inferiorly and placed carefully in the superior surface by the use of correct surgical technique with the countersink drill is likely to integrate favourably. By contrast an ill-defined open weave pattern in the anterior maxillae with little cortical bone in the superior surface or nasal floor may offer little security for the fixture (**4.51**). When this is found to be the case during the operation, the possibility of using a larger diameter fixture within the bony canal may exist in order to provide stability, i.e. 5 mm exchanged for a 3.75 mm diameter. Such a solution does not exist with a narrow jaw.

Failure to secure firm anchorage in cortical bone for the fixture is likely to result in ineffective osseointegration. The surgeon may therefore need to warn the patient before operation of the uncertainty in placing implants in such situations where radiographs indicate the volume and quality of bone are poor (**4.52**).

Examination of study casts

Patient assessment leading to planned treatment

- Medical and dental histories
- Clinical oral examination
- Radiographic examination
- Possible psychiatric opinion
- Articulated study casts
- Evaluation of trial dentures/diagnostic wax up
- Agreed surgical plan/template for surgery
- Discussion of options/agreed treatment plan
- Signed consent form

Case planning, including the design of the implant prosthesis, requires the preparation of well-made study casts and their correct mounting upon a suitable dental articulator.

When assessing the edentulous case, it is necessary to prepare trial, conventional prostheses and validate both the jaw relations and the tooth arrangement. Where suitable dentures exist, the trial arrangement may be created from a duplication of the existing set. The casts should be marked to identify from the radiographic evidence the anterior positions of the antra and the incisive fossa in the maxillae. In the mandible, the cast should be marked with the positions of the mental foramina. The possible implant sites, separated by the width equivalent to the fixture diameter e.g. 4 mm minimum, can be marked on the jaw surface. Five or six are usually chosen in the anterior edentulous mandible for a fixed prosthesis (**4.53**). Two to four may be chosen for a complete overdenture prosthesis. Where doubt exists about the relation between the potential arch and the implant sites because of their location or inclination, then either the artificial teeth in the trial set-up may be indexed, removed from the trial denture and inspected or a wax duplicate may be poured and substituted for the denture. Wax may then be cut away from the base so that the required direction of the fixtures can be judged. Using this approach, both the surgeon and the prosthodontist can evaluate the ideal fixture positions and angulations (**4.54**).

Evaluation of the partially edentulous case is even more critical. A diagnostic wax-up of a fixed prosthesis or trial arrangement of artificial teeth will confirm for the patient what the likely outcome, including its shortcomings, may be and precipitate a properly argued discussion about surgical and prosthetic goals (**4.55**). It is particularly important to correlate evidence from study casts, clinical findings and radiographs since the predicted evidence of the quantity of bone may allow the surgeon to have viable options that avoid subsequent restorative problems. It is therefore often useful to site replica components into the casts in order to ensure that a required position for the fixture will place an abutment correctly in the intended arch and in relation to the natural dentition. This is especially important with a deep incisor overbite, for example.

Study casts should be marked with the position of each fixture and be made available with a surgical template to assist the operator to insert fixtures (**4.56**). Templates are prepared from the diagnostic wax-up or from a wax duplicate of the trial denture. Part of the template must be capable of being properly stabilised on the teeth or upon the uninvolved mucosa (**4.57**). It is necessary to consider four factors when designing the template. These are: access to the operative site, the need to place a mouth prop during anaesthesia, room to retract the mucoperiosteal flap and clearance to position the components at the fixture sites (e.g. direction indicators). A commonly used design is to create the labial aspect of the intended arch of the prosthesis to ensure that access to future abutment connections lie within the arch (**4.54**). A template with channels for the guide bur or twist drill is most useful in preparing the bony canals but this design makes the assumption that bone exists in the correct volume diagnosed in the examination of the patient's case. Where extremely accurate positioning of the fixture is required, i.e. in depth and angulation to ensure the correctness of the position and shape of the prosthesis, the surgeon may be advised to have a labial and lingual template of different design.

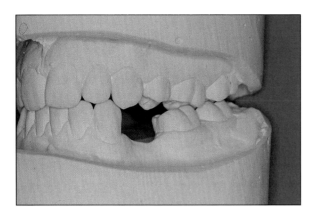

4.1 Does this space need to be restored? The decision must depend upon an assessment of risk versus benefit.

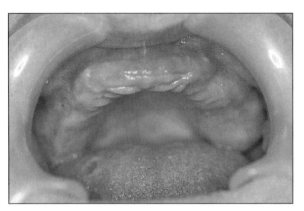

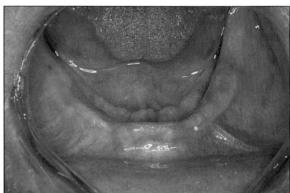

4.2 Good jaw ridges suitable for conventional complete denture construction.

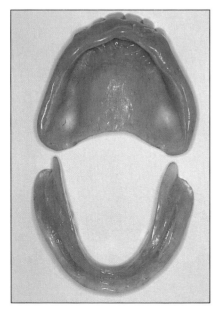

4.3 Alternative treatment with complete dentures in preference to implant-stabilised prostheses.

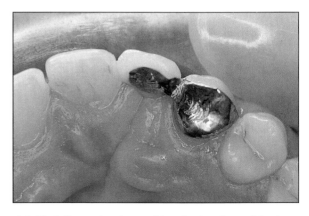

4.4 Cleft lip and palate with missing lateral incisor replaced by a resin-bonded bridge.

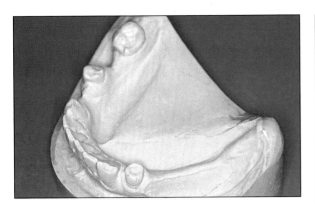

4.5 Dental cast showing multiple saddle areas, including a narrow ridge more suited to restoration with a distal extension removable partial denture.

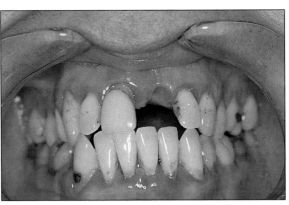

4.6 A site of single tooth loss in a neglected dentition displaying recession of the gingivae and gingivitis.

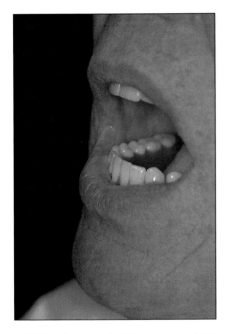

4.7 Displacement of lower complete denture poorly controlled by the patient.

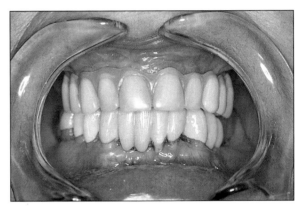

4.8 Intolerance of dentures evoking severe retching has caused the patient to seek preservation of the dentition together with implant treatment leaving the palate exposed (bridge made by the patient's own dental surgeon).

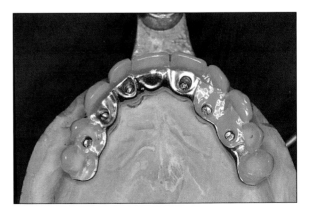

4.9 The maxillary fixed prosthesis leaving the palate free from coverage.

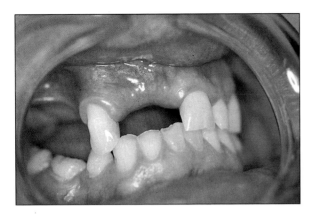

4.10 Dentition displaying tooth surface loss due to parafunction in a medically compromised patient. Case unsuited to implant treatment.

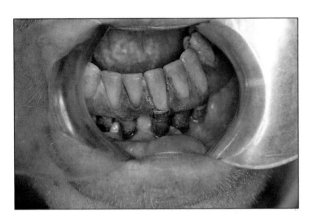

4.11 Failed treatment resulting from neglect arising from a depressive illness associated with alcoholism.

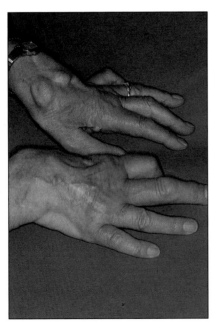

4.12 Physical limitations imposed by rheumatoid arthritis may impair cleaning so prejudicing the standard of oral hygiene.

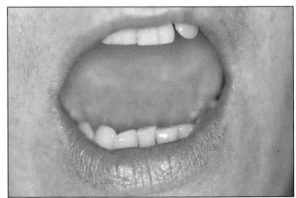

4.13 Maximum gape showing limited inter-incisal clearance insufficient to permit access for instrumentation.

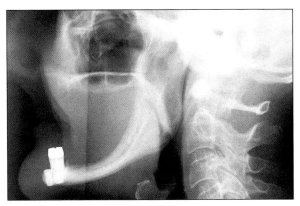 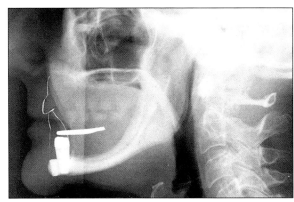

4.14 Loss of lip support associated with extensive maxillary resorption. Lateral skull X-rays indicate the need for flanges. (Radiopaque markers are placed over the central incisor teeth.)

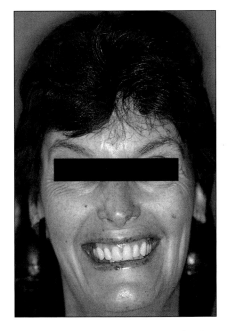

4.15 Short upper lip allowing display of the flange when smiling.

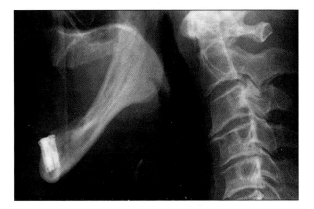

4.16 Adverse jaw relations making implant treatment difficult.

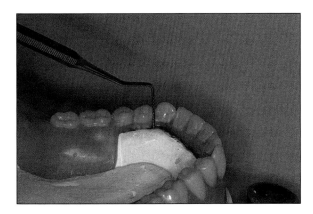

4.17 Assessing the space for components using trial dentures.

63

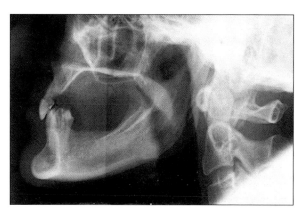 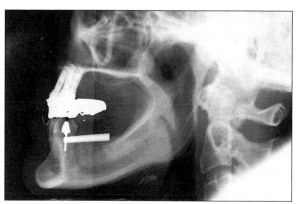

4.18 Conflict of alignment of the dental arch and alveolar ridge. Lateral skull X-rays show the dentition and its replacement with a fixed maxillary prosthesis using angulated abutments.

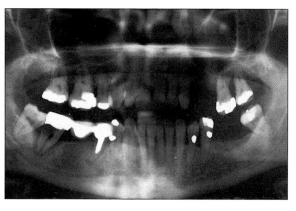 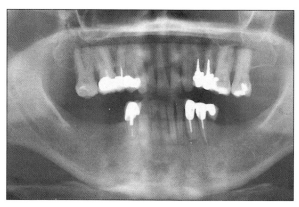

4.19 A failing dentition exhibiting chronic periodontal disease and a failing bridge resulting from periapical infection. Case unsuited to implant treatment.

4.20 Teeth of doubtful prognosis showing extensive restorations, unresolved apical disease and over-eruption of unopposed teeth.

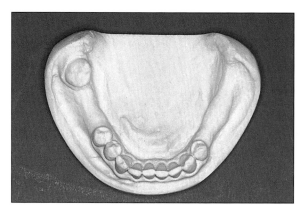 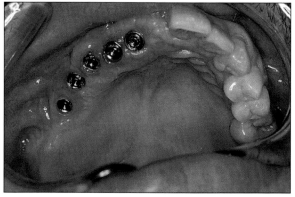

4.21 Typical example of the pattern of tooth loss where a partial denture has been discarded by the patient.

4.22 Long free end span suitable for implant treatment in maxilla.

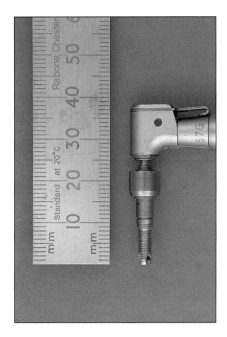

4.23 Drill, fixture mount and 10 mm fixture set against rule to identify the minimum gape and space between the operative site and the opposing jaw.

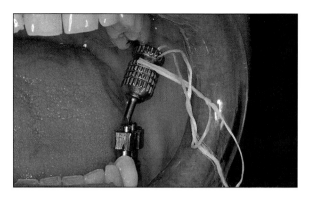

4.24 Limitation of space between posterior aspects of dental arch despite use of a short (20 mm length) screwdriver.

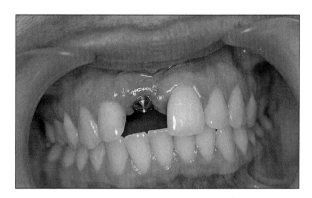

4.25 Loss of single tooth from an intact arch creating a span greater than one unit. A healing abutment is in position.

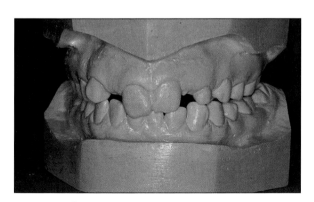

4.26 Arch spans apparently sufficient to accommodate a single unit in each space.

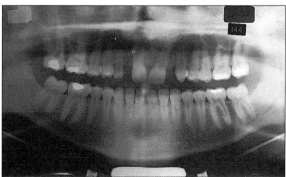

4.27 Radiograph showing an inadequate interradicular space to accommodate implants.

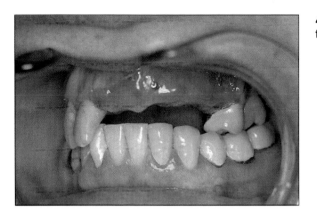

4.28 Long anterior span suitable for implant treatment (teeth lost in an accident).

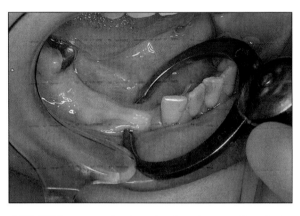

4.29 'Ridge mapping' under local anaesthesia to determine bone thickness.

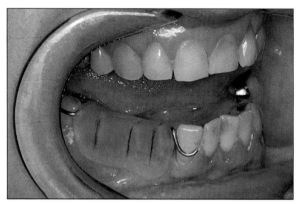

4.30 Template with metal markers to indicate proposed implant sites.

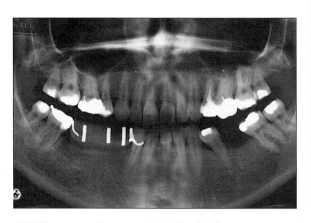

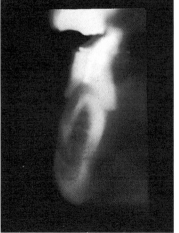

4.31 Tomographs recorded with the Scanora apparatus showing available height and width of bone to encompass implants at one of the selected sites indicated by the metal marker.

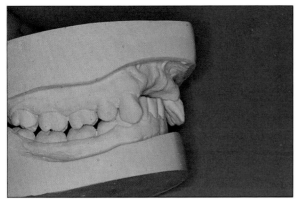

4.32 Study casts used to identify the placement of implants before operation. Alveolar resorption favours the use of a flange.

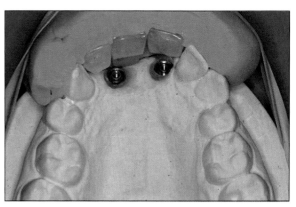

4.33 Replica abutments used to assess the restoration of this case complicated by a deep overbite.

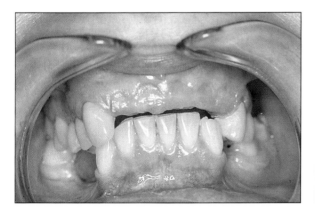

4.34 Deep incisor overbite restricting the use of implants.

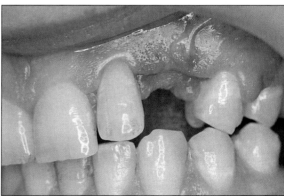

4.35 Local loss in a canine site complicated by over-eruption of opponent tooth and the risk of canine guidance disturbing the prosthesis.

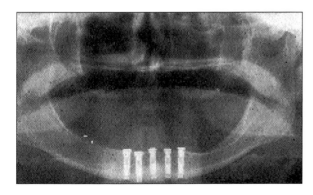

4.36 Favourable basal bone in the anterior mandible. Suitable for implantation.

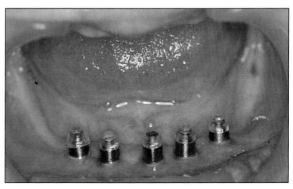

4.37 Poor intra-oral shape of mandible ('ridge') due to alveolar resorption in this case.

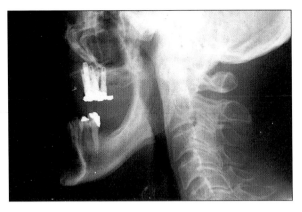

4.38 Severe malrelation of jaws.

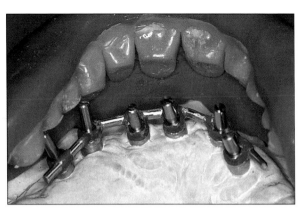

4.39 Cast showing implant solution with overdenture.

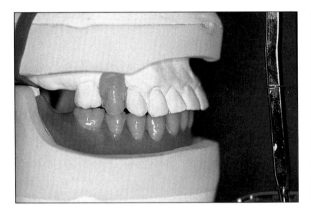

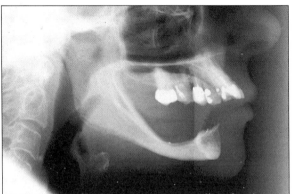

4.40, 4.41 Edentulous atrophic mandible opposed by partially dentate arch creating problems in cantilevering and in restoring the occlusion.

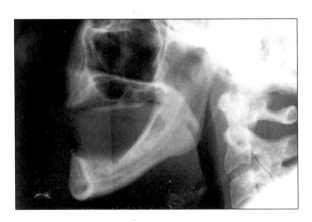

4.42 Sharp mandibular ridge offering poor support to a complete denture.

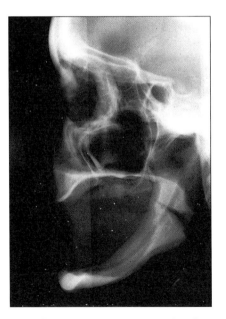

4.43 Gross alveolar resorption including the body of the mandible. Favourable shape of maxillae.

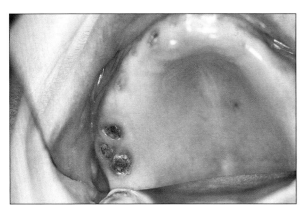

4.44 Clinical view indicating the presence of retained roots requiring extraction.

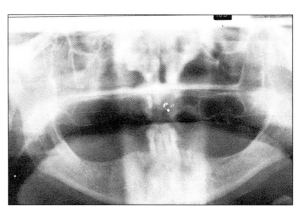

4.45 Radiograph indicating the presence of retained roots requiring extraction.

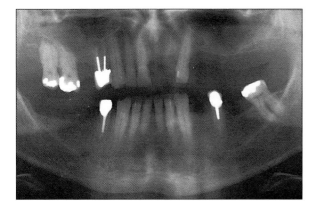

4.46 Large antra restricting the sites of available alveolar bone to the anterior maxillae.

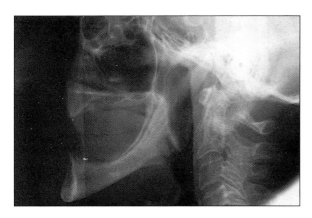

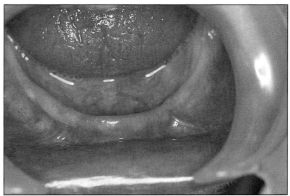

4.47, 4.48 Lateral skull radiograph and clinical photograph of the mandible with sufficient height but limited thickness.

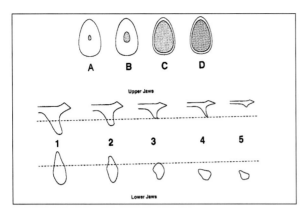

4.49 A classification of jaws indicating the potential quantity and quality of bone available for implantation.

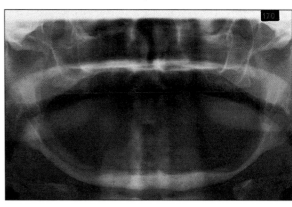

4.50 Minimum bone height available for shortest fixtures (7 mm) in case of advanced resorption of mandible. Augmentation should be considered.

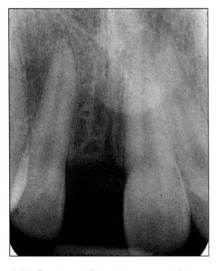

4.51 Poor quality open weave bone in site of missing incisor tooth.

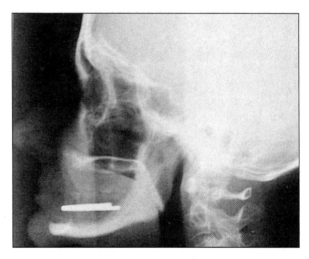

4.52 Dense residual bone in the anterior mandible contrasting with the poor quantity available for implants in the maxillae.

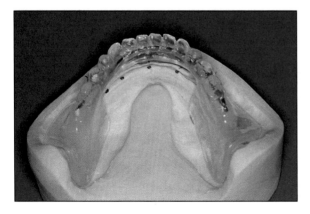

4.53 Surgical template prepared for locating fixtures for a mandibular fixed prosthesis.

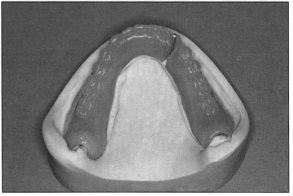

4.54 Diagnostic duplicate wax-up of a complete denture relating the potential position and direction of a fixture to the denture space.

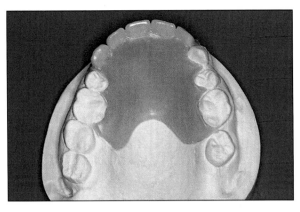

4.55 Partially edentulous case with diagnostic trial wax denture.

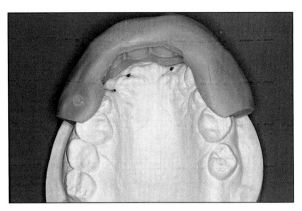

4.56 Teeth related in index showing planned implant sites on primary cast.

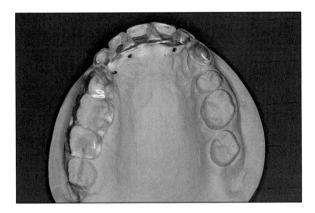

4.57 Template prepared for operation. Note one area is free to maintain access for a mouth prop if the operation is performed under general anaesthesia.

5. Implant-Stabilised Complete Overdentures

Introduction

Dentures that are stabilised by implants and may be removed by the patient are termed implant-stabilised complete overdentures. The retentive elements are housed within the fitting surface of the denture and attached to the abutment secured to the implant fixture (**5.1, 5.2**). The simplest system comprises either a ball and retaining cap, or a magnet and keeper located upon a single implant. Alternatively, two or more implants may be linked by a bar over which is placed a retaining sleeve or clip (**5.3, 5.4**).

This treatment is most frequently used for the stabilisation of complete mandibular dentures. In some situations extraction of natural teeth, rendering the patient edentulous, may result in a well-healed ridge, offering a favourable foundation to support and stabilise a complete denture that recovers for the patient a pleasing appearance, and the capacity to articulate clear speech and to chew most foods effectively. Both tolerance and acquired muscular controlling skills play an important part in the ability to wear dentures successfully. The acquisition of such skills is essential as resorption of the ridge occurs, gradually decreasing the support of the denture. However, advanced bone loss resulting from previous periodontal disease or the continuance of ridge resorption may result in a most unfavourable supporting tissue for the denture. Flat and inverted jaws (categorised as Zarb and Lekholm type 3 or 4, or Cawood and Howell III, IV, V or VI) demand great skill by the patient to wear and control the denture without discomfort.

The lack of success of treatment, using even well-constructed complete dentures, may be dramatically improved by positioning a limited number of implants (usually two in the mandible) which integrate with the jaw and so offer stabilisation of the prosthesis (**5.5, 5.6**).

An alternative viewpoint would consider the removable prosthesis to be a cheaper form of implant treatment to a fixed prosthesis that demands the support of a minimum of four fixtures integrated in the edentulous jaw. Apart from increased cost, the complete fixed prosthesis may prove unsatisfactory in design where the full extent of the occlusion is required (e.g. opposing an intact dentate arch) and the required position of the arch is so buccally placed to the dental supporting tissues (so-called ridge) that a flange is

necessary. This is especially so in restoring the correct contours of the lips and cheeks. Likewise the display of abnormally positioned long crowns or titanium abutments will spoil the appearance of those patients who reveal the mucosa when smiling or speaking (i.e. those patients with high lip lines). In limited numbers of patients complaints are made of degraded speech with escape of saliva and air above maxillary fixed prostheses and below mandibular fixed ones. The alternative use of complete overdentures may eradicate these difficulties.

The number of implants placed in the jaw is usually from two to four, all or some of which may be activated to stabilise the overdenture (**5.7, 5.8**). In the mandible it is common practice to position one in each canine or first premolar area and one or two spaced in the incisor area (according to the size of jaw), which remain as inactivated reserve fixtures in case of failure or subsequent loss of integration. Mandibular bone is usually dense with a good thickness to the inferior cortical layer. Hence mandibular implants are readily stabilised in the anterior jaw surface. By contrast, the texture of the maxillae is often poor with an open weave pattern and little cortical bone. The volume of available bone in resorbed jaws is much less, so that the resorbed maxillae are significantly more difficult to treat.

Few prospective studies of the outcome of overdenture treatment followed over a 5-year period have been published. Early data would seem to imply that short length (7 mm and 10 mm) fixtures may be used successfully only in the mandible (**5.9–5.11**). In treating the maxillae it is suggested that 13 mm or longer fixtures should be used, especially in the canine buttress. It is preferable to use at least two implants on either side of the incisive foramen in the jaw (**5.12–5.15**). The need for grafting bone in cases of severe resorption and any improvement that may follow from increasing its volume is not yet clear. Many techniques have been described but long-term data are not available.

Overdentures should be designed to sound prosthetic principles with maximum functional coverage of the edentulous jaw to gain optimum support and stability. Correct jaw relations with an increased freeway space of 2–4 mm between the premolar teeth should be created, together with a tooth arrangement producing a balanced occlusion and adequate facial support. It is not appropriate to reduce base coverage or create occlusal schemes that provide unbalanced eccentric tooth contacts. In these circumstances, unstable dentures will unfavourably increase the loads transmitted to the limited numbers of dental implants.

Debate exists about the ideal design of the anchorage between the prosthesis and the integrated implants. Since loads must inevitably be shared between the edentulous jaw covered by mucosa and the limited numbers of implants, it would appear logical to permit some movement of the prosthesis about the attachment to the implants, especially in the mandible. An increased number of implants, together with support offered by the palate to the denture, may make this less important in designing the anchorage of the maxillary prosthesis (**5.16, 5.17**). Leverage of the implants must be minimised and loads require to be directed from the horizontal occlusal table down the long axis of each one. In order to secure the optimum effect, the points of retention for the prosthesis should be positioned close to the jaw surface by avoiding the use of long abutments. Hence, where these are combined with cylinders to link the units with a bar, the combined height should usually not exceed the height of the supporting fixtures.

A commonly used design in the mandible is to position two fixtures in the canine area, to which are secured 4 mm or 5.5 mm abutments to carry 4 mm gold alloy cylinders. Soldered between the cylinders is a straight platinised gold alloy round or oval bar (e.g. Dolder pattern) to which is applied a clip or sleeve. This permits some (1 mm) vertical translation as well as rotation by the denture. For this to occur there must be relief in the prostheses over and around the cylinders and the abutments. There should also be clearance for the leaves of the sleeve so as to enable it to function (**5.18–5.21**).

Improvement in the mechanical stability of the denture may be provided by extending two cantilever arms distally in the line of vertical rotation. An additional distal clip may then improve the resistance to vertical withdrawal. Cantilevers less that 8 mm are recommended, but it is not clear if this design is mechanically sound from the viewpoint of implant loading. It is important that the clips lie in the same vertical path of insertion (**5.22**).

Linkage of the cylinders with a curved bar as opposed to a cranked design is unlikely to permit rotation and both will increase leverage upon the implants (**5.23**).

A common alternative solution is to position individual ball anchorages on two isolated implants. Various designs are available with different implant systems based on the concept of the Dalbo stud, developed as a radicular precision anchorage. The low profile of the Nobelpharma stud forming part of the abutment unit is advantageous in reducing the height of components in relation to both the fixture length and the space required in the prosthesis. Although exact parallelism is not essential, deviations greater than 20° are likely to increase the seating forces and stress at the implant–bone interface when the denture is inserted or removed.

Improved denture stability may also be gained from magnets acting upon titanium-coated keepers screwed to isolated implant abutments. The inevitable make and break created by small movements of the denture leads to wear of the surfaces of the keeper and magnet, producing loss of the protective coat and ultimately possible corrosion. A fundamental problem exists where the occlusal loads applied to the denture cannot be transmitted to sufficient numbers of implants. A sharing of loads between the edentulous jaw ridges and the magnets cannot be achieved without displacement of the denture pivoting around the keeper. While some patients consider such dentures are improvements, others complain of the lack of firm contact and repeated sounds of make and break between the magnets and keepers.

Retention for the maxillary prosthesis should naturally exist from border seal. Stability is enhanced by using non-resilient joints between either round- or parallel-sided bars fully engaged by sleeves or clips.

Anchorage for overdentures
• Stud and cap
• Keeper and magnet
• Bar and sleeve/clip
• Cone and coping

Designs of joint
• Rigid
e.g. Parallel bar with matched sleeve
• Resilient
e.g. Round bar with spacer and clip

A comparison of complete implant-stabilised overdentures with complete dentures

- Stability and retention is increased by anchorage from implants in resorbed jaws.
- Comfort in wearing a complete implant-stabilised denture avoids using a resilient lining.
- Improved resistance from implants to buccal and labial forces may improve tooth positions in the dental arch.
- Facial support from denture flanges is maintained in complete overdentures.
- The occlusal table of the complete overdenture may oppose all teeth in the opposing arch (i.e. natural dentition).
- Efficient cleansing of components and the mucosal cuff will require the patient to exert good standards of prosthetic care and oral hygiene.
- Load sharing with the implants will require regular monitoring and correction for loss of support due to edentulous ridge resorption.
- The frequency of denture adjustment including rebasing and replacement is unlikely to be significantly less for implant-stabilised dentures than complete dentures.

The provision of treatment

The decision by the oral surgeon and prosthodontist to provide a complete implant-stabilised overdenture will be made when a fixed implant prosthesis is impractical due to cost or limited availability of bone, and where the patient prefers to have a removable prosthesis. It must be clearly understood by the patient that a successful outcome will be dependent on regular maintenance and monitoring and that the benefits will be different from a fixed prosthesis (**5.24–5.25**).

Radiographic examination using lateral skull and orthopantomographic views should indicate if it will be possible to place implants (in the canine and incisor regions) only in a severely resorbed mandible (**5.26–5.29**). Often tomograms of the maxillae will be required to identify if there is sufficient volume of available bone.

Well-made articulated study casts set up with trial dentures should be available (**5.30, 5.31**). Examination of the distance in the anterior mandible between each mental foramen in comparison with the trial denture will suggest the most suitable positions in which to site a straight bar

between two implants. Where the available denture space is in doubt, a wax duplicate of the denture will allow channels to be cut in the line of the planned fixtures to confirm their direction in the chosen positions. The bulk available for future components between the jaw and the denture surface can also be explored (**5.32, 5.33**).

When a decision upon the number, size and position of the implants is reached, a clear acrylic resin surgical guide (template) can be constructed from a duplicate of the trial denture to aid the surgeon in implant placement during the first operation (**5.34a,b**).

The lower implant-stabilised complete overdenture offers the surgeon a good way to start using the osseointegration technique.

A comparison of complete implant-stabilised overdentures with complete fixed prostheses

- Total retention and stability is created for the fixed prosthesis which is screwed in position by the dentist. A complete overdenture that is removable by the patient exhibits small amounts of movement during function.
- Facial support offered by the extension and width of the flange of the complete denture covering the resorbed ridge cannot be achieved by a fixed prosthesis.
- The fixed prosthesis reduces the volume of the space required by the overdenture in the oral cavity, with the potential to improve tolerance.
- A reduction in the length of the occlusal table and restriction of the amount of cantilevering of the dental arch away from the implants is required by the fixed prosthesis.
- Cost will be less of providing a complete overdenture with fewer components than a fixed prosthesis.
- It is more demanding of the patient to achieve the required standards of oral hygiene whilst cleaning a fixed prosthesis.
- Partial transfer of loads to the edentulous ridge by overdentures may promote resorption and necessitates greater frequency and volume of treatment to sustain the occlusion and fit of the overdenture (**5.24, 5.25**).

Clinical examination should answer a number of questions:

- If the jaw is resorbed is there sufficient width (minimum 5 mm) and depth (minimum 7 mm) to accommodate suitable implant fixtures?
- Is the zone of attached mucosa of the supporting tissues narrow? This will result in the probable exit of abutments through a mobile cuff which may create difficulty in establishing mucosal health?
- Are there unfavourable structures within or adjacent to the denture base? (For example, mandibular tori, sharp prominent mylohyoid ridges and genial tubercles which may compromise the mandibular base. Thick fibrous tissue covering maxillary ridges will compromise the cuff surrounding an abutment and may require surgical reduction.)
- Is the denture space occupied by the patient's existing denture abnormal? (For example, a narrow anterior space may be dictated by the form and behaviour of the investing lips, cheeks and tongue. The angulation of the fixture and the exit of the abutment will need to be determined precisely.)
- Is the jaw relation abnormal? (A large 'inter-ridge' space between the surfaces of the jaws will increase the volume of the prosthesis and the potential leverage upon the dental implants.)
- Is the occlusal relation unfavourable? (If one jaw is edentulous and the other dentate, the relationship with the natural teeth may preclude achieving a balanced eccentric occlusion.)
- Will the difference between the position of the jaw 'ridge' and the likely artificial tooth position create a major disparity? (Abutments, cylinders and bar components may increase the bulk of the anterior palate of the denture base.)
- Is the existing denture well-designed and capable of being modified to accommodate the implant components? (Less than ideal designs will require the replacement of existing dentures. For example, denture bases should offer sufficient support to the occlusion. The arch form should adequately support the face.)

Surgical management

Predictable surgical preparation of bone that would allow repair and encourage acceptance of a biocompatible foreign material inserted into it was systematically evaluated by Brånemark in the early 1950s. Subjected to a scientific appraisal, the appropriate restraint was built into the design and use of suitable instruments and the Brånemark (Nobelpharma) Implant System was commercially launched in the early 1980s; many other systems have been developed since.

Surgical technique

All of the currently used implant designs necessitate meticulous and ordered surgical technique. The surgical procedures are most often completed under local analgesia with or without intravenous sedation but can be performed under full nasotracheal intubation with obturative throat packing. Infiltration of a local anaesthetic into the labial and lingual sulci is in any case an advantage to provide perioperative haemostasis and post-operative analgesia. The recommended technique for the Brånemark system utilises a labial sulcus incision made approximately 1 cm from the crest of the ridge (**5.35**).

Caution should be exercised in the atrophic jaw as nerve fibres from the mental nerve may arise not far from the crestal bone and accordingly should be identified and retracted. The mucoperiosteal exposure is deepened through the bellies of the mentalis muscles and then, in the subperiosteal plane, the flap is reflected lingually to reveal the whole superior surface of the anterior mandible between the mental foramina. This, in the grossly atrophic jaw, may be diminutive in size. When the lower jaw is atrophied it will probably be perforated through the lower cortical margin to secure implant stabilisation. This is a painful experience for the patient unless the cervical and submental nerve supply have been dealt with locally. Knowing the likelihood of purposeful perforation, submental infiltration in the sulcus should be used in advance of the surgery.

Lingual flap reflection allows a broad-based, well-nourished flap to repair where the suture line does not coincide with implant position. Exclusion of the implant site thus reduces the chance of continuing contamination of this critical area during the initial healing period. It also replaces intact periosteum with regenerative power over the implants.

Influence of local anatomy

On occasion, reflection of the mucous membrane presents a bony architecture that is inadequate for implant placement, i.e. it is too thin antero-posteriorly or is everted at the crest and undercut below. Such a ridge will require vertical reduction, resulting in removal of cortical bone from the superior border. Placement of a fixture in cancellous bone most often leads to bone loss next to the shoulder and loss of implant stability during the subsequent healing phase. Shallow cortices should be preserved with allowance made for the fixture to seat whenever possible in the cortex. With atrophy, the bone bulk reduces in three dimensions but largely at the expense of the alveolus and eventually the basal bone. Thus the vertical dimension of the jaw is reduced.

Thin mandibles have hollows lingual to the lower lateral incisor areas and lingual soft-tissue retraction will demonstrate that bony format. Hence adequate depth of the jaw may not always be accompanied by sufficient width in the residual ridge.

Bone resorption often leads to a reduced distance between the mental foramina. Awareness of the position of the mental foramen is necessary to avoid permanent nerve anaesthesia or paraesthesia.

Volumetric reduction of available mandible creates a need for use of the inferior border by the fixture. Bicortical stabilisation (even with 7 mm fixtures) accordingly offers rigid stability for overdentures. Tenting of the periosteum inferior to the mandible allows bony in-filling around the projecting fixtures in these cases.

Mandibular resorption leaving an inverted pattern with a high lingual plate or high genial tubercle will lead to implant placement that will require appropriate clearance in the design of the overdenture. Technical difficulty with implant placement adjacent to an inclined plane created by the jaw shape may lead to thermal trauma of the bone, particularly at the countersink stage. It may also lead to exposed threads on either the lingual or labial surface of the implant.

Basal bone texture is often more dense than alveolar bone. This produces more resistance to the cutting instruments and accordingly more thermal trauma. In these cases it is important to drill slowly and carefully, with copious coolant.

Plentiful irrigation of all cutting instruments reduces the frictional element and accordingly the heat rise. The need to reduce temperature rise to below 47°C is adhered to. Animal studies have confirmed that temperatures in excess of 47°C, especially when achieved for periods in excess of one minute, damage bone and encourage its repair with fibrous tissue. Whilst there are differences in cutting sequences between different systems in the preparation of channels to receive implants, the general principles are similar. Here, the Brånemark system will be described.

The exposed mandible allows perforation sites to be chosen for a small number of implants. The location of these sites will be aided by a template that allows the surgeon to appreciate the future contours of the planned denture. The implant alignment should preferentially allow the long axis to be lingual to the dental arch and within the denture space. Excessive lingual inclination will increase the bulk against the tongue; conversely a fixture placed too far labially may lie outside the labial flange and the implant abutment will subsequently impact against the lip. In a small mandible, three implants are placed; a more voluminous bone may support four. Only two of these will subsequently be used and the others allowed to lie dormant and to act as 'spares' should fixture failure occur at a later date.

Surgical progress

Surgical stages in osseointegration

SURGICAL STAGE 1
- Preparation of bony canal
- Insertion of implant fixture
- Application of cove screw

INTERVAL FOR HEALING
- 3—6 months, dense bone (mandible)
- 6 months, less dense bone
- 0 months, both stages together but delay loading/restoration

SURGICAL STAGE 2
- Exposure of implant head (local flap or punched channel)
- Removal of cover screw
- Attachment of healing abutment

POST-OPERATIVE HEALING OF MUCOSAL CUFF

A rose-head bur perforates the superior cortex of the visible mandible passing into the cancellous area below. It provides immediate information to the surgeon about bone texture (**5.36**).

This is then followed by a 2 mm twist drill rotating at up to 2000 revolutions per minute (rpm), with the torque set to drive in the shaft to the appropriate depth. The shaft is marked with depth indicators so that the channel may be sequentially enlarged to a matching dimension. Copious irrigation at the time of insertion takes cooling saline along the twist drill to the cutting site and withdrawal of the drill while still rotating brings out the bone dust with the saline irrigant. The drill is inserted and withdrawn without widening the aperture (**5.37**).

Completion of the channel to the chosen depth then allows a pilot drill to be inserted. This instrument allows a 2 mm width to be enlarged to a 3 mm diameter (**5.38**). At this stage, assessment of the direction of the channels may be made by temporarily siting direction indicators. Alteration of the direction of the hole may be made (**5.39–5.42**).

With little jaw height, purposeful perforation of the lower border is completed. There is always increased resistance as the twist drill passes through and control must be maintained during this manoeuvre. The channel is prepared to the chosen depth according to markings on the twist drills. Some implant systems involve spade-like instruments that gouge bone. These are passed to the appropriate depth and form the definitive shape of the implant. This allows a rigid fit of the implant into the prepared site with digital pressure.

The discussion as to whether mucous membrane should be repaired over the implant continues. The arrangement recommended by Brånemark is that the incision should not coincide with the implant to avoid contamination, and to allow for periosteal placement over the fixture. Initial stabilisation provides the optimum arrangement for acceptance of the implant, and Nobelpharma and other threaded implant systems encourage screw tapping the channel in the bone to increase the surface area of titanium available for osseointegration (**5.43, 5.44**). This also provides immediate stability. This procedure is completed by motor with a rotational speed of about 12 to 15 rpm. Reversal of the tap is done cautiously. The prepared channel is measured for usable length and a fixture, untouched and uncontaminated by contact with gloved fingers or other metal, is driven into the site, copiously irrigated and hand cranked home (**5.45, 5.46**). The Brånemark implant shoulder should be in cortical bone. A cover screw is next inserted to protect the central screw hole, the hexagonal-shaped top of the fixture lying slightly proud of the bone surface (**5.47**). Almost all implant designs provide a cover facility. Failure to seat the cover screw may encourage soft tissue or even bone to grow over the shoulder of the implant and even up to the hexagonally shaped top. Removal of this bone may result in damage to the implant.

Difficulty in seating the cover screw sometimes occurs when the countersink has not cut the opening of the canal in the line of the long axis of the implant fixture. This is more likely to occur, for example, when the bone surface is shelved and a thick close lingual cortex guides the countersink incorrectly into a labial tilt.

Debridement of the wound should be completed, especially in the lingual periosteal fold. The mucoperiosteal repair is effected in the sulcus with vertical interrupted 4/0 catgut sutures to allow for mild mucosal eversion and a slight post-operative ooze. There is absolutely no indication for non-resorbable suture materials to be used – a variety of materials being available that have varying resorption times.

Pressure for 15 minutes over the wound is followed by administration of the appropriate antibiotic therapy and post-operative analgesia regime. It is advisable to defer immediate denture placement. After wound closure, mucosal relief for 10 days is advised. Subsequent adjustment and a reline of the existing denture with functional impression material will resist preferential masticatory loading of the cover screw sites (**5.48**). Transmission of masticatory force to a prominent cover screw is tantamount to the fixture being loaded, which may deter osseointegration. Early relief of any soreness by appropriate prosthodontic treatment is indicated. Pain occurring after implant placement is most commonly due to a loose cover screw.

The second surgical stage will be timed by the surgeon according to the clinical condition he meets at installation. Thin or hardly recognisable mandibular cancellous bone may encourage a six-month delay before the second-stage surgery. Similar concern about integration in poor quality bone may encourage an even longer wait when treating the maxillae.

Presurgical radiography frequently confirms integration but films occasionally do not confirm failure. This is detected later when the cover screw is removed or when the abutment is added. Obvious looseness of the implant or its rotation in bone indicates a lack of integration. Other diagnostic features are a dull percussive note when the abutment is struck or even pain when the cover screw is undone.

The second surgical stage is also preceded by local infiltration and, on occasions, mandibular block anaesthesia. If the fixtures are very superficial then the cover screws can often be seen through the mucous membrane. Accurate trephining with a mucosal punch allows simple and rapid dissection of the disc of tissue that displays the underlying screw. It is in fact rare that the trephine neatly punches the full thickness of mucous membrane. The hexagonal shape of the implant superior surface is then exposed by removal of the screw and the shoulder cleared to its periphery. This is difficult to do through a small aperture. Crestal incision through preferably keratinizing epithelium, over the full extent of the jaw housing say three or four implants, will allow mucosal reflection lingually and labially. Direct visibility of the implants and their cover screws permits subsequent clearance of all soft tissue and bony regrowth from each of the implant sites.

Bone clearance from the hexagonal implant surface must be done without damaging the fixture.

Some implant systems provide healing abutments that are slightly larger than the size of the definitive transmucosal abutment (TMA) to be placed when the mucosa has healed. This facilitates treatment by allowing the operator to remove the healing abutment, to see the hexagonal or other entrance site of the fixture and to place the appropriate length of transmucosal component accurately after measuring from the surface of the fixture top (**5.49**). Experience has shown that a three-week period of healing between the exposure stage and the definitive measurement for a transmucosal abutment provides a stable partially epithelialised tract. Mucosal repair should wrap the mucous membrane closely around the TMAs, and the neater the repair the shorter the time between surgery and reconstructive phases of treatment. When definitive abutments are placed at the second operation they are sealed with healing caps retaining a periodontal dressing under them and the patient is returned to the prosthodontist.

Pain experienced after placement of a transmucosal abutment is most commonly due to a loose component.

Special considerations for maxillary implant-stabilised overdentures

Generous maxillary width and height allows very straightforward implant placement. For overdentures, no less than 10 mm of bone height is needed to support implants. Mucosa incision for the placement of implants at Stage 1 is made in the labial sulcus approximately 1 cm from the alveolar crest. Palatal reflection of the mucous membrane usually spares the incisive bundle and fixture siting will be according to prosthetic demand and template design. Fixtures placed in the canine/premolar region will be desirable. Maxillary implant placement is usually quicker than in the mandible and often the self-tapping technique is used in which the appropriate fixtures create a threaded channel in the softer, less dense bone. It is important that engagement of the cortices of the nasal floor or the anterior wall of the antrum is achieved to resist the insertion/withdrawal forces used in seating or removing the prosthesis and those inflicted upon loading of the overdenture during mastication and by bruxing habits.

Purposeful use of the 2 mm twist drill to reach the nasal floor and enlargement with the combined twist countersink instrument can be completed very rapidly using the self-tap technique. Caution should be exercised, however, where the crestal bone of the maxilla is narrow when using this cutting tool or if its use is contemplated near to a thin cortical plate. Rotational forces may pull it through a weak wall. In this situation, it is advisable to use the conventional 3 mm twist drill followed by a countersink, but this does not subsequently preclude the use of a self-tapping fixture.

Mucosal thickness in the palate is variable and may require careful contouring, following attachment of the abutments, to avoid deep mucosal cuffs which inhibit effective cleansing of the sites. Furthermore, excessive soft-tissue coverage will demand the use of long abutments which, together with the cylinder, increase the potential for leverage on short fixtures.

Post-operative management

Approximately two weeks after the insertion of the implant fixtures, the mucoperiosteum is sufficiently healed to allow the existing complete denture to be reinserted, restoring the appearance and function of the patient. In order to avoid undue loading of the healing mucosa and, more importantly, the newly inserted implants, the anterior surface of the denture base should be reduced to provide a 2 mm clearance of the mucosa. A visco-elastic lining is then applied to the dry denture surface and the prosthesis is inserted to allow the material to be moulded. Surplus material is removed before the patient is discharged and asked to return after a week to check the result. The lining will require to be replaced at appropriate intervals (usually two or three times in 4–6 months) if it hardens, becomes rough or indicates pressure over the implant sites.

After the second surgical operation to place the abutments, the mucosal cuff will usually be sufficiently healed within 10 days to allow the denture to be fitted over the healing abutments. Either the denture may be coated with a thin wash of alginate impression material or the abutments are marked with a tracing pencil, so that on insertion it is clear where the contact between the two hinders the appliance from being seated (**5.49**).

A tungsten carbide denture-trimming bur or steel bone bur can be used to penetrate the visco-elastic lining and, if necessary, the base, to create the desired depressions in the lining material. A small addition of fresh material will ensure an exact fit, creating for the first time a sense of stability for the denture (**5.50, 5.51**).

In the absence of swelling and oedema, a primary impression is made using, where available, the existing special tray constructed for the interim complete denture (**5.52**). However, if a satisfactory interim denture with a correctly extended base has already been achieved then it may be duplicated using silicone putty to produce a cast for the construction of an acrylic resin special tray and a poured-wax record block. Whichever approach is used, it is essential to appreciate that the (custom) special tray should be made to a correct extension to produce the most favourably supported and stabilised denture, unlike the tray made for a fixed prosthesis. On the primary cast, two exit holes are outlined within the tray border to allow passage for the transfer copings that will be placed for this procedure (**5.53, 5.54**). Acrylic trays are normally designed with finger rests and a small extending sleeve around each hole, in order to secure stability for the material surrounding the impression copings. If the interim denture is unsuitable in design then a correctly made stock tray impression is required to produce a primary cast.

A well-made working impression may be recorded using a stiffly set elastomer (e.g. polyether impression material). Before making the impression, the prosthodontist should position the tray and adjust the extension by tracing with compound or by shortening the borders.

Topical anaesthetic is applied to the healed mucosa cuff before removing the healing abutment. Since the size of this component is already known, a suitable exchange with a conventional TMA may be made which places the top of the abutment at the mucosal surface or, preferably, 1–2 mm superior to it. (**5.55**). The precise position is determined by the ultimate length of the components in relation to the fixture length, and the space available for the dental arch and body of the overdenture. For example, a 7 mm fixture would be at risk to unfavourable leverage if a 5.5 mm TMA and 4 mm cylinder were added. When securing the abutment screw of the Nobelpharma system it is appropriate to use 20 N/cm torque in an electric torque controller.

Having checked the accuracy of fit of the abutment (using a long cone technique for an intra-oral X-ray if necessary), the transfer impression coping may be attached using a long fixing screw. For securing the impression coping, gentle pressure sufficient only to prevent rotation of the coping is obtained with a hand-held screwdriver.

When both copings are in place, the tray is lowered to ensure easy seating with sufficient clearance for the impression material (**5.56**). The tray is dried and a tray adhesive applied and allowed to dry. A thin wash of mixed material is applied with a spatula up to and including the tray border and the tray is inserted (**5.57, 5.58**).

The mandibular impression is properly made by encouraging the patient to raise the tongue during insertion of the tray. When it is correctly seated, controlled border movements are produced by the patient – the prosthodontist having previously rehearsed these actions with the patient. The completed impression should record the supporting tissues for the denture base in a displaced form. The oral mucosa of the bearing tissues, with the exception of the cuff around the abutments, should then contribute to support provided by the implants.

When the material is set, the impression is released by unwinding the fixing screws. The impression is washed for one minute and a decontaminant antiseptic spray used to minimise the risk of cross-infection to the laboratory.

Abutment analogues are secured with the fixing screws to the copings (**5.59, 5.60**). The impression is boxed and poured in modified die stone. Ultimately another cast should be poured, the first for reference and the second for fabrication of the denture.

The jaw relations may be recorded using a temporary resin base and wax occlusion rim, which is prepared to fit over the replica abutments upon the master cast (**5.61, 5.62**). Alternatively, a closer representation of the already planned jaw relation can be achieved by first adapting the fit of the duplicate denture to the master cast and then using it to make the recordings. This has the major advantage of replicating the desirable design features of the existing denture.

Assuming the existing maxillary denture is satisfactorily designed, a duplicate alginate impression may be made to pour a replica cast in stone. Also a transfer facebow recording is taken to locate this cast to the hinge axis of the articulator.

With both casts mounted and the articulator programmed (set with the appropriate values) the complete overdenture may be set up for trial insertion in the mouth (**5.63–5.65**). After validation and approval by the patient, the trial arch should be indexed using either Plaster of Paris or silicone putty so that the positions of the incisors, canines and first premolar teeth may be assessed in relation to the replica abutments. Excessive prominence of the dental arch, anteriorly and superiorly to the resilient joint formed between the denture and the planned components providing the retention, may indicate revision of the tooth positions in order to reduce the unfavourable effect of the denture tilting about the bar when it is subjected to incisal loading. Likewise, close proximity between the arch and abutments may provide inadequate space for these components. A limited space, reducing the bulk of acrylic resin over the components, may also dictate the construction of a cast strengthener for the prosthesis.

Two gold alloy cylinders are positioned upon the replica abutments and a resilient form of bar cut and soldered to them using an investment technique that allows sufficient solder to form an adequate union with the cylinder and bar (**5.66–5.68**). Since the bar (and sleeve) must lie within an adequate volume of the prosthesis, some variation in its position or the use of cranking may become necessary. It is usual to assess the exact fit of the bar and cylinders to confirm the accuracy of the impression before proceeding to finish the denture.

In the laboratory, the sleeve is positioned over the bar using a 1 mm spacer. The trial denture is cut away to provide 2 mm clearance around the cylinders and the sleeve (including its retentive element). A 1–1.5 mm thick coating of Plaster of Paris is now applied to the cylinders and to the inferior aspects of the sleeve as well as the zone below the bar (**5.19, 5.69**). When complete, the trial denture is rewaxed, sealed to the cast and invested. Conventional packing, processing, divesting and polishing techniques are used to finish the denture. Split cast mounting may be employed to refine the occlusion before divesting the cast. However, it is appropriate to remount all cases with a precontact check record in order to ensure that the occlusion is correctly balanced in the intercuspal position (**5.70, 5.71**). Finally, the sleeve may be adjusted to ensure optimum retention. Failure to block out the cylinders and the sleeve will not allow a resilient joint to function (**5.72, 5.73**).

Complaints by the patient of inadequate retention may arise because of incorrect laboratory technique or inappropriateness of this design. Inexperience with the laboratory technique may result in inadequate seating of the denture over the joint. Improper blocking out over divergent cylinders or around the sleeve will be found. Disclosing wax placed in the base and in the sleeve will reveal if the denture is correctly seated. Acrylic resin may be trimmed away to rectify these faults. When the mandibular incisor and canine teeth are positioned well in front of the resilient joint, the patient may complain of dislodgement of the denture during incising food. Similar complaints during chewing can occur if the bar is diagonally positioned due to the original misplacement of the implants. For example, this occurs if one fixture is positioned in the premolar site and another in the lateral incisor region on the other side of the jaw. This problem may be overcome by activating a third fixture in the mid-line of the jaw or by extending distally the anterior bar with two extensions so providing additional clips to limit the displacing movements created by incision or chewing sticky foods.

Alternative technique: rebasing the existing denture

When a simpler system of anchorage is to be used, an existing well-designed complete denture can be modified to incorporate the female component. For example, the healing abutment may be exchanged with an abutment retained by a gold alloy ball anchorage screw (Nobelpharma system 3, 4 or 5 mm height). The plastic retaining cap (5.4 mm diameter, 4 mm length) is positioned upon the male unit and the fitting surface of the denture is fully relieved to allow the denture to be seated. Undercuts are also removed from the base. When using a medium-bodied addition cured silicone wash impression material, an adhesive is applied to the denture surface first; otherwise, a thin coat of zinc oxide eugenol impression paste is used and the denture is seated. Border movements mould the impression, which is allowed to set whilst the teeth are in maximum intercuspation. In order to secure an accurate relation between the retaining cap and the denture, it is important to unite it using a self-curing resin linkage with the denture base, after the impression has set. The denture is withdrawn and a laboratory component replicating the male anchorage is fitted into the retaining cap. The impression is boxed and cast. An index relating the denture to the cast is also made prior to removing the denture. Before rebasing the denture in a conventional way, a 0.8 mm height spacer is applied to the laboratory abutment replica and screw so that the repositioned plastic cap will be raised to a position that will allow vertical translation or rotation about the ball anchorage.

It is of course possible to make the impression using transfer impression copings positioned upon the abutments provided the denture base can be perforated without damage to the artificial teeth in the arch (i.e. there is a lingual relationship between the implants and the lower arch).

Construction of complete maxillary overdentures

The techniques for producing maxillary overdentures which are stabilised by implants are very similar.

A special tray precisely covering the support tissues is required. If there is any doubt about the length of abutment to be used it may be more helpful to use transfer copings screwed to the fixture heads rather than those which attach to the regular abutments. A choice may then be made of the abutment height in the laboratory. An open-top box rather than individual openings for the passage of the copings may be designed, provided this does not interfere with the recording of the true sulcus shape by over-extending the border of the tray. Replica components are screwed to the transfer copings retained in the completed impression before the cast is poured.

An accurate recording of the jaw relationship is followed by a trial insertion which is approved by the patient. It is now possible to examine more precisely the choice of components and their positions in relation to the intended polished surface contours of the denture. For example, the arch and polished surfaces may be indexed with silicone putty, both on the buccal and on the palatal/occlusal surface, in order to relate the surfaces to the cast. The teeth are removed from the trial denture and set into the index without the temporary base. Examination of the space which is seen to be available in both the vertical and horizontal directions will reveal the limit of the height of abutments and gold alloy cylinders, as well as the position of retaining bars and clips. Arbitrarily increasing the palatal thickness to accommodate the components may result in complaints by the patient of poorly articulated speech. A choice between a precision bar with clips (e.g. Dolder system) or a laboratory cast and milled bar incorporating precision attachments (e.g. Ceka) is commonly made. (Magnets with keepers have the advantage of occupying less space but maintenance problems exist with some systems.)

Follow-up and maintenance

> **Follow-up for complete overdentures**
> - Check for balanced occlusion
> - Assess retention of joint
> - Confirm fit/border extension
> - Examine fit of denture over components
> - Check screw retention

It is essential to have a regular programme of follow-up and maintenance to ensure the success of treatment and avoid damage to the mouth (5.74–5.78). The patient will require instruction in both denture cleansing and efficient use of Superfloss and interdental brushes to cleanse both the cuffs and the abutments and attachments. It is easier to maintain good oral hygiene than with fixed prostheses, since the denture is removed for cleaning and fewer, more widely spaced, implants

are employed. When the mucosa is sore to brush, hyperplasia of the cuff is more likely. A similar response below the bar usually indicates failure on the part of the patient to remove the denture at night, thereby encouraging stagnation of plaque.

The abutments and cylinders linked by screws should be examined for tightness at one week and one month after fitting, in order to check for looseness. This is less likely when an identifiable correct torque is applied with a torque controller. The small gold alloy screws are more prone to failure than abutment screws. Where failure of osseointegration is suspected, the bar should be removed and each component checked for security.

Retaining clips and sleeves will require adjustment to tighten them at yearly intervals. However, early dissatisfaction with the stability created by the joint may indicate that it is not activated, has been abused by the patient biting the denture into place, or that a fault exists in the design of the denture, typically an over-extended flange or unbalanced occlusion. Often the experienced patient will exert adequate control over the stabilised overdenture even when the clip has lost retention upon the bar.

After a more prolonged period of wear, resorption of the jaw or abrasion of the artificial teeth will promote denture ulceration. Tooth replacement on adequately fitting dentures is possible. A loss of fit will require the prosthodontist either to rebase the denture or remake it. On most occasions it is easier to remake the prosthesis using a duplication technique, especially when a bar joint is used. The existing bar is most conviniently removed and placed on the replica abutments in the new cast after a successful trial insertion, in order to position the sleeve.

> **Protocol for case management**
> - Patient history
> - Assessment of articulated study casts and diagnostic trial prosthesis
> - Discussion and agreement of treatment options and preferred plan withj patient
> - Stage 1 surgery — implant insertion (3—6 months healing period)
> - Stage 2 surgery — healing abutment connection (2—4 week healing period)
> - Prosthetic treatment, including permanent abutment connection
> - Planned recall and maintenance
> - (Problem solving)

SUMMARY OF THE PROSTHODONTIC TREATMENT PHASES OF COMPLETE LOWER OVERDENTURE STABILISED BY DENTAL IMPLANTS

Phase 1: Record primary impressions
- Recorded over healing abutments or after exchange with permanent abutments.

Phase 2: Position permanent abutments
- Remove healing abutment from healed cuff.
- Measure depth to fixture head.
- Select permanent abutment in order to project surface 2 mm above the cuff.
- Locate abutment with 20 N/cm torque.
- Add healing caps.

Phase 3: Design special trays
- Ensure correct coverage for support.
- Provide access for impression transfer copings.

Phase 4: Record master impressions
- Remove healing caps.
- Attach impression transfer copings with long or short fixing screws.
- Insert special tray, check fit and extension with sufficient clearance for copings.
- Apply adhesive, record elastomeric impression with correct border moulding procedure.
- Remove impression and replace healing caps.

Phase 5: Pour master casts
- Screw brass replica abutments to transfer copings.
- Box and pour impression in stone.

Phase 6: Design record blocks
- Outline base, wax out undercuts on cast.
- Prepare light cured acrylic resin base with access for fixing screws.
- Add wax rim.

Phase 7: Record jaw relations (including transfer face bow record)
- Select teeth.

Phase 8: Trial insertion
- Set up teeth into balanced occlusion.
- Confirm jaw relations after removing healing caps.

- Examine facial support offered by arch and flange relative to a stable position of the denture.
- Index the try-in on the master cast.

Phase 9: Prepare the resilient joint
- Position 4 mm gold cylinders with fixing screws on brass replicas.
- Measure and cut length of resilient bar to be positioned 2 mm clear of mucosa.
- Check clearance with teeth using the index.
- Unite bar to cylinders with Duralay resin, ensuring adequate wrap around.
- Invest and solder the bar to the cylinders.

Phase 10: Try-in the bar joint
- Confirm each cylinder has a passive, exact fit upon the titanium implant.

Phase 11: Prepare denture for finishing
- Locate cylinders on laboratory replica abutments.
- Position spacer and sleeve upon bar.
- Cut back trial denture and seat on cast to confirm clearance.
- Remove denture and plaster out relief upon cylinders, on sleeve margins and below bar.
- Reseat and seal denture.
- Finish denture.

Phase 12: Insert completed dentures
- Remove healing caps, check abutment screws.
- Secure cylinders with gold fixing screws using 10 N/cm torque.
- Insert denture and record check record to remount case. Refine occlusal balance.
- Reinsert denture. Check sleeve retention.

Phase 13: Record long cone X-rays to show marginal bone level

Phase 14: Reassess dentures
- Examine components including security of the gold screws.
- Monitor oral hygiene standard.

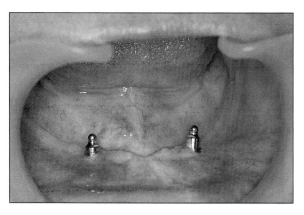

5.1 Astra abutments carrying retaining studs.

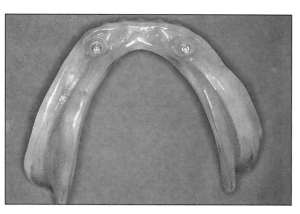

5.2 The fit surface of denture showing individual retaining Astra caps.

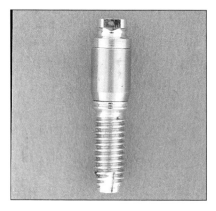

5.3 Brånemark implant, abutment and gold alloy cylinder used for bar/sleeve joint.

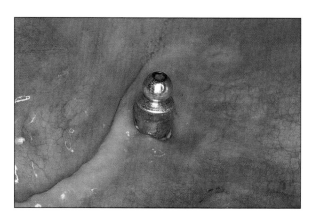

5.4 Implant abutment and ball anchorage, substituting for the cylinder.

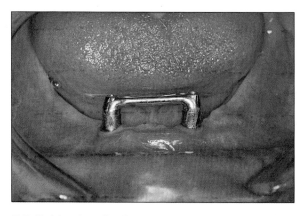

5.5 Dolder bar linking two cylinders secured to abutments placed five years previously.

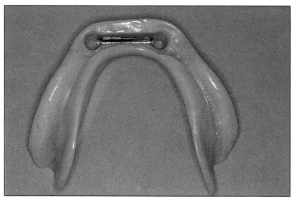

5.6 Fit surface of complete implant-stabilised overdenture showing a well-extended base and a retaining sleeve.

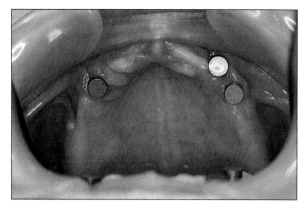

5.7 Edentulous maxillae with limited available bone used to house three functional implants with keepers screwed to the abutments.

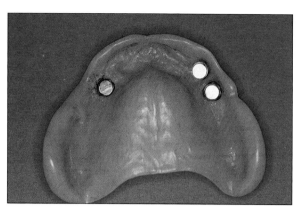

5.8 Complete maxillary overdenture enclosing three rare earth magnets.

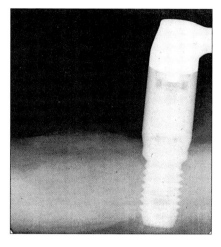

5.9 Periapical radiograph showing fixture in atrophic mandible engaging the inferior cortex.

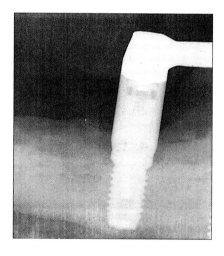

5.10 Three and a half years later the fixture remains fully functional with no evidence of bone loss.

5.11 Periapical radiographs showing favourable fixture length compared with the combined abutment and cylinder lengths.

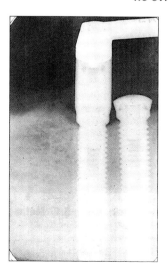

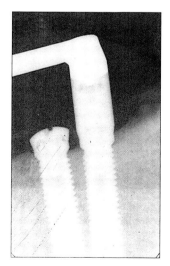

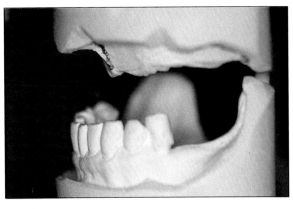

5.12 Study casts showing an unfavourable Class III jaw relationship.

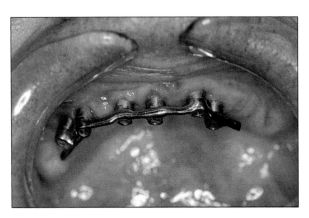

5.13 Edentulous maxillae showing multiple implants linked by a Dolder bar.

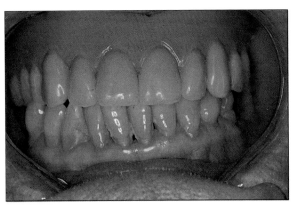

5.14 Overdenture *in situ*.

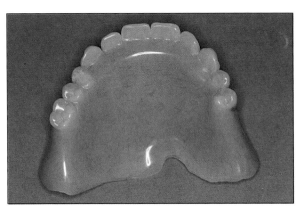

5.15 Palatal contour of the overdenture.

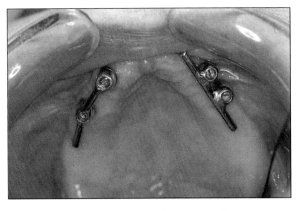

5.16 Lateral bars providing retention for an overdenture in the maxillae.

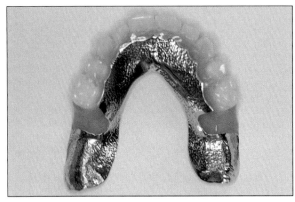

5.17 Metal-based overdenture prepared for the case.

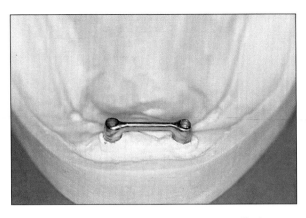

5.18 Completed Dolder bar soldered to cylinders.

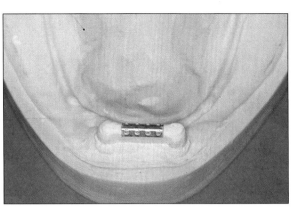

5.19 Sleeve located on a spacer over the bar with the cylinders and retaining edge of the sleeves masked with Plaster of Paris.

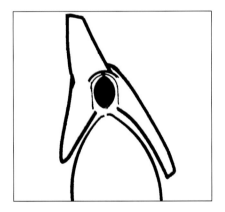

5.20 Cross-sectional diagram of the bar and sleeve correctly located in the denture space.

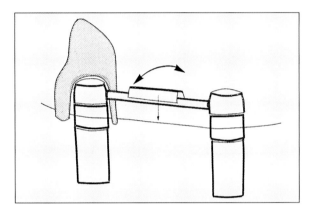

5.21 Diagram illustrating the potential movements of the stabilised overdenture.

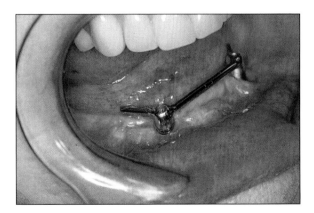

5.22 An oval bar with two cantilever extensions offering more stability.

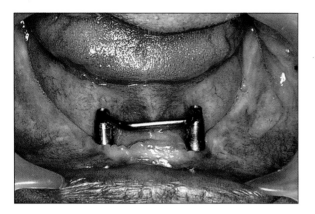

5.23 A cranked bar is required because of the unfavourable distal placement of the right fixture in the premolar region.

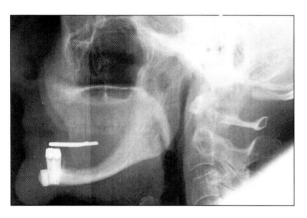

5.24 Lateral skull radiograph showing the implant-stabilised overdenture *in situ* after five years.

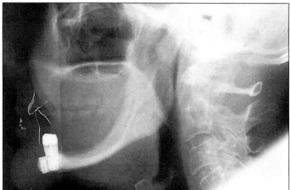

5.25 Radiograph showing the corrected jaw relations and the improvement in the facial profile with the replacement prostheses.

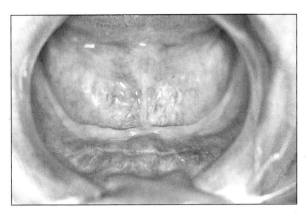

5.26 Edentulous mandible of a patient complaining of repeated soreness and looseness of the lower complete denture.

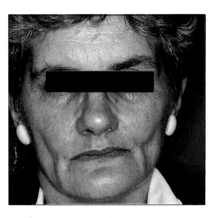

5.27 Loss of facial support in the absence of complete dentures.

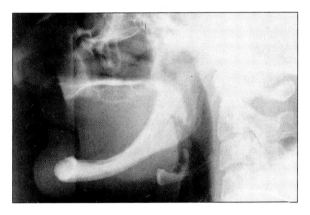

5.28 Skull radiograph showing the extent of resorption of the jaws. Sufficient height exists in the anterior mandible to accommodate fixtures of approximately 10 cm in length.

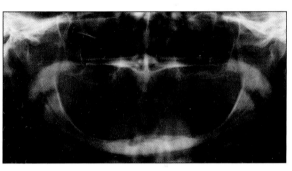

5.29 OPG radiograph of edentulous jaws identifying sufficient depth of bone in the anterior mandible.

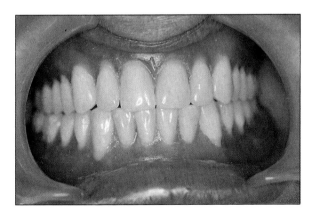

5.30 Trial complete dentures prepared for case assessment.

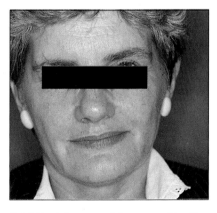

5.31 Facial support improved by the trial complete dentures of the patient in 5.27.

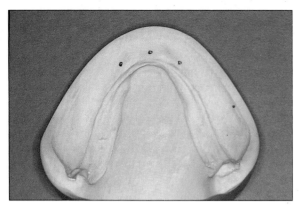

5.32 Study cast prepared from a primary impression of the jaw, marked to show three potential implant sites.

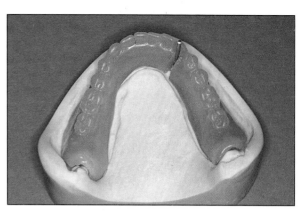

5.33 Duplicate of the trial complete mandibular denture poured in wax to allow the position and direction of a planned implant to lie within the denture space.

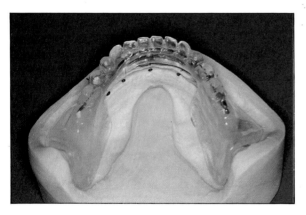

5.34a Surgical template prepared for locating fixtures for mandibular fixed prosthesis.

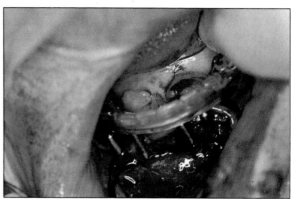

5.34 Template in use. One canal is misaligned with the arch, lying too far buccally.

Surgical sequence of treatment

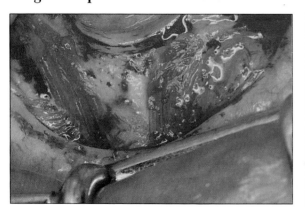

5.35 Incision made in the labial sulcus one centimetre from the ridge crest.

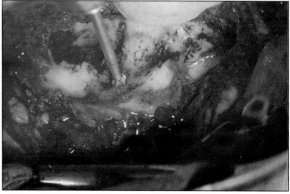

5.36 Penetrating the cortical surface with a rose-head bur to identify the site of a bony canal.

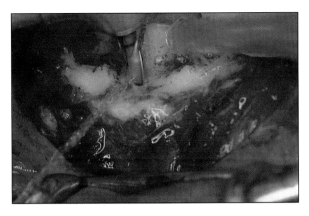 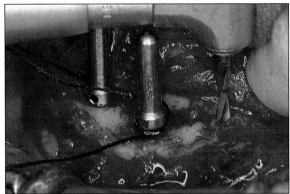

5.37 Use of a twist drill to deepen the penetration of the bone. (Two canals have already been prepared.)

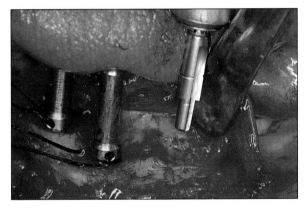 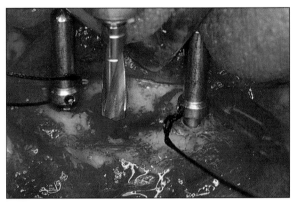

5.38 Enlargement of the orifice of the canal with a pilot drill.

5.39 Confirming the direction of the canal with an indicator. Insertion of a 3 mm twist drill.

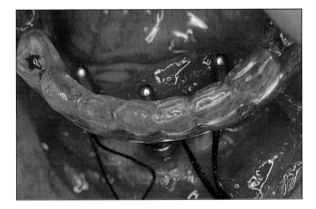 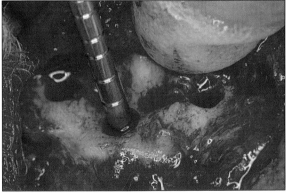

5.40 Examining the relationship of the canal to the denture space by means of a surgical template.

5.41 Measuring the depth of the canal with a graduated gauge.

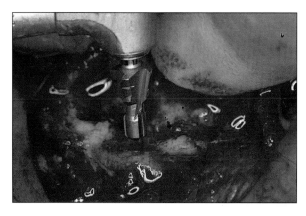

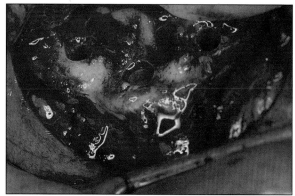

5.42 Applying a countersink drill to enlarge the orifice to accept the fixture head.

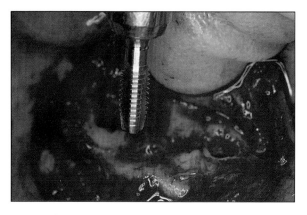

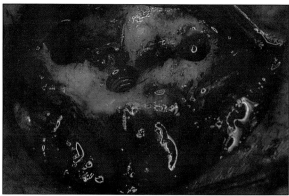

5.43 Using a titanium tap to impart a thread to the canal surface.

5.44 The area of surface contact with the titanium fixture is enhanced by the cut threads.

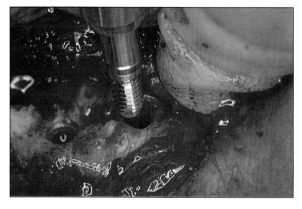

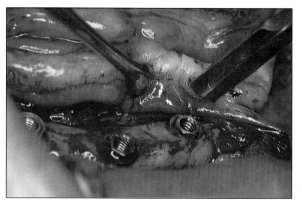

5.45 A titanium fixture secured to a mount positioned within the handpiece coupling.

5.46 The fixture *in situ*.

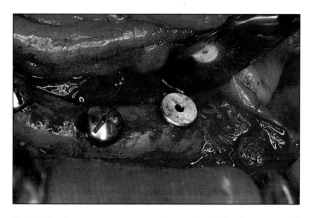

5.47 Placing a cover screw to protect the hexagonal surface of the fixture.

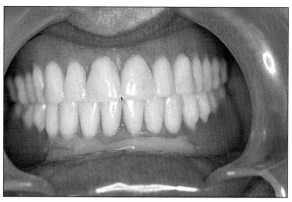

5.48 The application of a temporary resilient lining avoids the risk of trauma to the mucosa and upon the implant fixtures after the surgical operation.

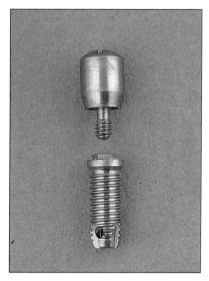

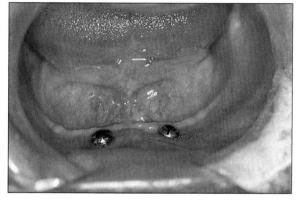

5.49 Healing abutments placed at the second surgical operation may be marked with a tracing pencil to localise the sites of relief for the complete denture.

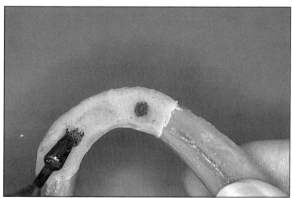

5.50 Penetrating the resilient lining with a steel bur.

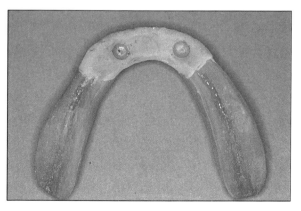

5.51 Temporary lining showing imprints of abutments which begin to create stability for the existing denture.

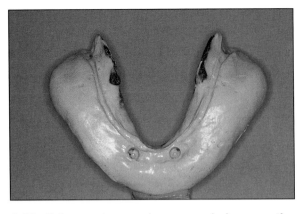

5.52 Primary impression recorded over the abutments.

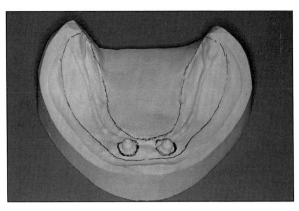

5.53 Primary cast outlined for a special tray.

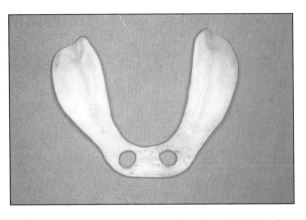

5.54 Special tray prepared with access holes for transfer impression copings.

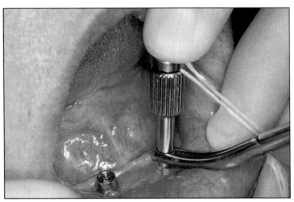

5.55 Exchange of healing abutment with permanent standard abutment.

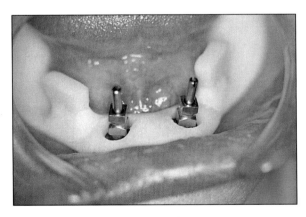

5.56 Trial insertion of impression tray.

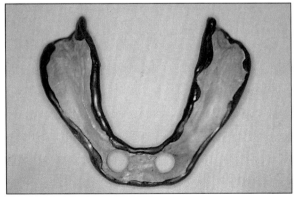

5.57 Border tracing of the tray.

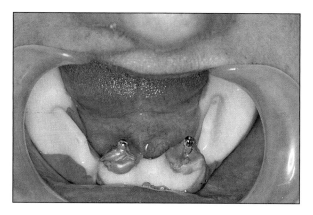

5.58 Completed impression.

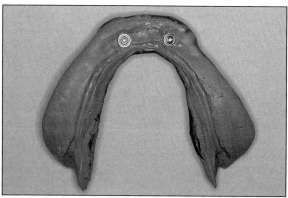

5.59 Completed impression ready to receive the dummy abutments.

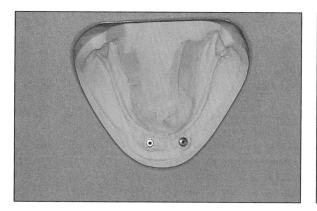

5.60 Master cast incorporating dummy abutments (brass analogues).

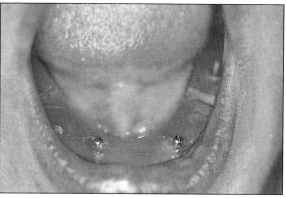

5.61 Conventional occlusion rim made on resin base, secured in the mouth.

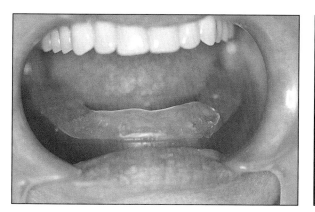

5.62 Upper trial denture opposing lower rim.

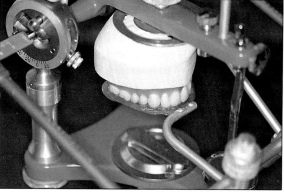

5.63 Mounting upper denture on the articulator.

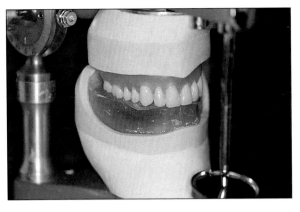

5.64 Mounted casts.

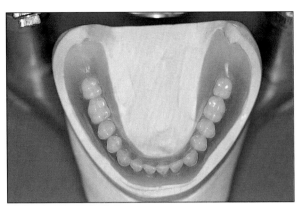

5.65 Trial arrangement of mandibular complete overdenture.

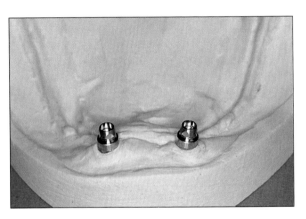

5.66 Two gold alloy cylinders to which a Dolder bar will be secured with 'Duralay' resin.

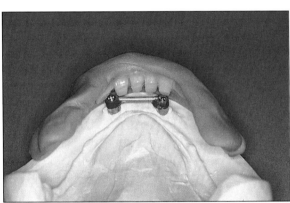

5.67 Silicone putty index used to check the intended position of the arch with the bar and cylinders.

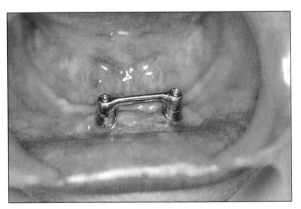

5.68 Dolder bar screwed to the abutments.

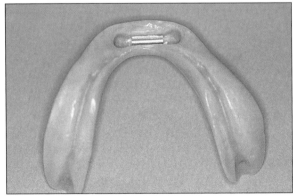

5.69 Completed mandibular overdenture showing the retaining sleeve and space to accommodate the cylinders.

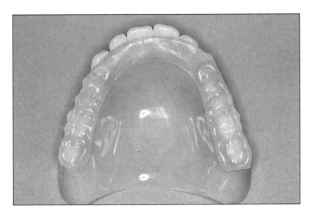

5.70 Pre-contact, occlusal check record.

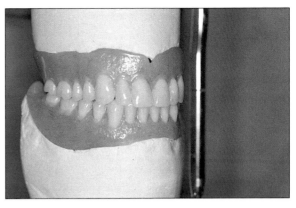

5.71 Balanced occlusion established in the retruded contact position.

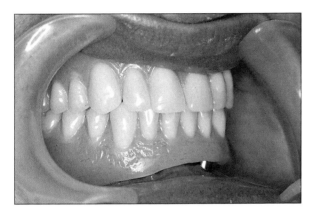

5.72 Completed dentures *in situ*.

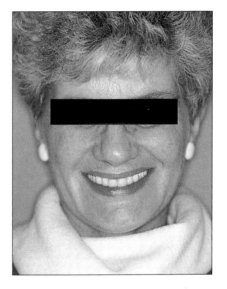

5.73 Facial support provided by dentures.

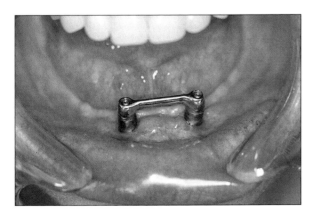

5.74 Case reviewed after an interval of one year.

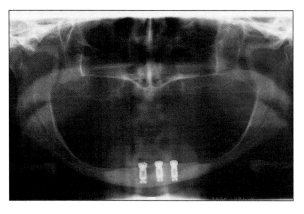

5.75 Three implant fixtures in the anterior mandible after stage one (OPG X-ray).

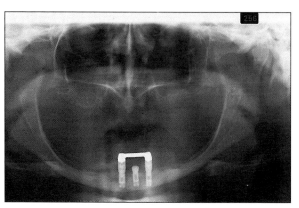

5.76 One implant fixture remains in reserve with a cover screw in place. Two fixtures carry standard abutments to which are attached gold alloy cylinders linked with a Dolder bar.

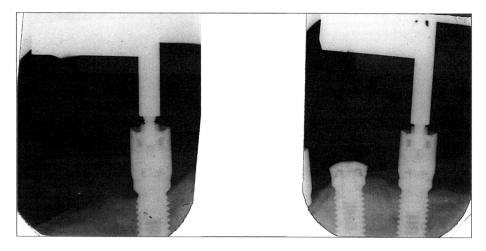

5.77 Intra-oral radiographs using a long cone paralleling technique to monitor the bone levels.

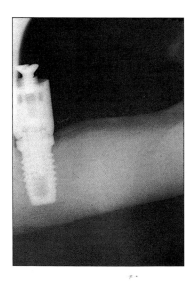

5.78 Intra-oral radiograph used to check the fit of the abutment on the fixture in another case. Notice the components are incorrectly mated and require the abutment to be reseated on the hexagonal top of the fixture.

6. Implant-Stabilised Fixed Prostheses

Introduction

The decision to treat patients with an implant-stabilised prosthesis should be based on a detailed assessment of their needs and the various treatment options available, as discussed in Chapter 4. Either a fixed or removable superstructure may be chosen; which is selected may be influenced by the patient's wishes or dictated by anatomical considerations. Although removable prostheses are often perceived by patients and clinicians as being inherently inferior to fixed superstructures, this is not necessarily the case, and either may provide superior performance in some situations.

The illustrations accompanying this chapter predominantly show treatment with a maxillary prosthesis, although a mandibular appliance is also shown. Construction of both mandibular and maxillary fixed prostheses follows exactly the same principles. Indeed the treatment carried out in the edentulous mandible recorded over 25 years indicates very high success rates for integration of implants in the anterior mandible and for the longevity of the cantilevered fixed implant-stabilised prosthesis. Four important considerations must be evaluated in planning such treatment:

- **Bone anatomy.** Is there sufficient depth and width of suitable bone to accommodate four or five fixtures?
- **Prosthesis space.** Is the pattern of bone resorption mild, thus avoiding the need for a flanged prosthesis to offer lip support whilst providing adequate room to accommodate a superstructure?
- **Fixture siting.** Are the potential locations of fixtures compatible with the positions of the teeth required to restore the appearance and occlusion without creating excessive leverage?
- **Occlusion.** Will the opposing prosthesis or natural teeth influence the choice of restoration?

Where less than a satisfactory volume of bone exists, it is necessary to make a decision either to provide an overdenture or to consider grafting the jaw or using guided tissue regeneration techniques to enhance the residual bone.

In an edentulous patient at least four, and up to six, fixtures will be required to support a fixed superstructure. The number depends on:

- **Implant length.** Longer implants can support greater forces.
- **Implant location.** Spaced implants are better able to resist the leverage which results from masticatory loads on a cantilevered superstructure than those grouped closer together.
- **Implant orientation.** Implants set around the curve of an arch are better able to resist tipping forces from a range of directions than are those set in a relatively straight line.
- **Bone quality.** The quality of the bone around an implant affects its resistance to loads. Where this is lacking in bulk and density then loads should be reduced.
- **Cantilevering.** Whilst loads on implants arising from forces applied directly between two fixtures cannot exceed the applied force, where distal cantilevers are employed much greater forces can be generated due to leverage. Shorter cantilevers should therefore often be used in the maxilla where osseointegration is usually less certain. Cantilevering effects also arise where teeth are placed buccally to the ridge.

There are, however, many other factors influencing the choice of a fixed or removable superstructure; these are summarised in **Table 6.1**.

Whilst the decision as to which type of superstructure to employ is made primarily on the basis of clinical examination and assessment of a trial or diagnostic denture, it is wise to caution the patient that, even with careful assessment, the findings at implant insertion may dictate the number and location of the implants which can be inserted, and hence the type of prosthesis which may ultimately be used.

Pre-surgical procedures

The final decision as to the type of superstructure to use will include the assessment of a trial denture, with the teeth arranged so as to satisfy the patient's wishes with regards to appearance, and the operator's requirements for an appropriate occlusal scheme and a superstructure design which will permit effective oral hygiene. Satisfactorily constructed complete dentures also form a good basis for planning the fixed prosthesis. The denture is duplicated and articulated against a cast of the opposing prosthesis or dental arch. Teeth are then set up, usually exchanging the second premolar for a molar tooth, and the denture indexed on the model to show the relationship of the teeth to the land areas. Having removed them from the duplicate denture, they may be repositioned in the index to contrast the position of the arch with that of the ridge. It is now possible to judge the preferred angulation and position of the implants. Any realignment of the teeth to correct a large potential discrepancy between the fixture sites and the arch should be carried out. The trial denture should then be duplicated in self-curing acrylic resin and trimmed to provide a surgeon's guide (template). A suitable design for the upper jaw is shown in **6.2**.

The important features of the guide are that it does not interfere with the surgical procedures and may be securely located, whilst providing enough information as to the positions and angulation of the implants. The guide should then be sterilised either with ethylene oxide or by soaking in an appropriate chemical agent, such as gluteraldehyde.

The patient's existing complete denture should be checked to ensure that it can be modified after surgery without fracture. If this is likely, then the denture should be strengthened in the region of the implant sites at this stage. If the denture itself is inadequate, then consideration should be given either to rebasing it or to making a temporary replacement.

It should be noted that, as a general principle, it is unwise to embark on implant treatment for a patient who already has an unsatisfactory denture until it has been replaced with a more suitable design and the outcome evaluated. A number of patients can be helped adequately by this means, whilst for those who are not, the new denture provides a model for a surgeon's guide, as well as a better temporary appliance during implant therapy.

Implant insertion

The techniques for implant insertion when using a fixed superstructure are the same as those when employing an overdenture, and have been described in Chapter 5. However, the procedure is more demanding in terms of the positioning of the implants. This is because, when using an overdenture, the prosthesis is removed to gain access to the implants, whilst with a fixed superstructure, access is initially through the fixed bridge prosthesis with its reduced potential to accommodate misaligned fixtures. In addition, the spacing of the implants is critical if occlusal loads are to be widely distributed and the abutments masked by the teeth.

Table 6.1. A comparison of implant-stabilised fixed and removable prostheses in the edentulous jaw.

Feature	Fixed	Removable
Number of implants	≥ 4 Usually 5/6	≥ 2
Stability	Very high	Design-dependent, can be high
Tooth positions	Restricted by limitations on cantilevering	More versatile, although excessive cantilevering will increase instability
Soft-tissue replacement	Limited by cantilevering and hygiene considerations	Can be extensive, e.g. a complete denture flange
Anterior seal	Limited by need to facilitate oral hygiene	A seal can be produced as with a conventional prosthesis
Bulk	Can have minimal bulk	More bulky
Occlusal table	Size limited by restrictions on distal cantilevering	Can be extensive
Support	Only on implants unless linked to natural teeth	May be soft-tissue supported, more commonly mucosa and implant supported
Cost	Expensive	Cheaper, as fewer implants and precious metals needed, appliance cheaper
Maintenance (long-term data not available)	More expensive	May be less expensive
Oral hygiene	Access can be difficult	Usually simpler as access improved with appliance removed

Post-surgical procedures

Once initial healing has occurred the sutures may be removed if a non-resorbable type has been used, and the temporary prosthesis inserted. This will usually need to be modified with a tissue conditioner to ensure an adequate fit. It is essential that there is no undue pressure over the implant sites, as wound breakdown may then occur. A thin mix of alginate impression material placed inside the denture without the use of adhesive forms an effective disclosing medium when relieving the prosthesis. Enough material should be removed from the denture base to allow for at least 2 mm of tissue-conditioning material. The patient will then need to be seen at regular intervals to review the status of the denture. In some cases it may be preferable to fabricate a temporary denture or rebase the old one, rather than make repeated temporary modifications to an existing prosthesis.

The implants should remain undisturbed for a period of 4–6 months whilst integration occurs. The interval depends on the patient's age, the quality of the bone into which the implants were inserted and whether they were placed in the maxillae or the mandible.

The presence of integration can then be checked using intra-oral radiographs, although it should be remembered that such techniques can demonstrate only the profiles of the implants and not the degree of integration all around the device. Furthermore, the technique is not capable of resolving the necessary interfacial detail, and integration has to be assumed on the basis of:

- Absence of radiolucencies adjacent to the implant.
- Evidence of new bone formation around the implant.
- Absence of loss of crestal bone, producing a cratered appearance marginally.

At this stage the implants are exposed and a second component, the trans-mucosal abutment (TMA) added to connect it to the oral cavity. This may be joined to the implant either mechanically, usually with a screw, or by a dental cement. The latter is simpler, but does not allow for ready replacement. This topic is discussed further in Chapter 3. The definitive standard abutment usually seats on the fixture in a positive fashion, but as the junction cannot be seen directly it may be wise to record a suitable radiograph to confirm that the abutments are fully seated.

Following the placement of the abutments, there is often a change in soft-tissue contour as healing proceeds and the tissue become less swollen. It should be remembered that the vertical space between the ridge crest and the occlusal plane is required to accommodate a zone for hygiene as well as the superstructure (**6.68**). Long abutments may facilitate cleaning at the expense of appearance or encroachment on the occlusal plane. This can result in the occlusal table being placed too far from the ridge, or the superstructure having inadequate height. For these reasons, many implant systems include a temporary or healing abutment which can be placed on the fixture when it is exposed. This component is usually slightly wider than the definitive abutment and may have a scale of some type on its surface to enable the thickness of the adjacent soft tissues to be measured when selecting the final abutments. Alternatively, a special probe can be used for this (**6.78**) when exchanging the healing component.

Previous careful inspection of the original study casts articulated with the trial dentures, and comparison of the position of the healing abutments in relation to the adjusted complete denture, will provide useful guidance on the choice of the style and length of the definitive abutments. In a majority of cases the measured depth of the healed mucosal cuff plus 2 mm produces sufficient clearance beneath the fixed prosthesis.

Where jaw relations are abnormal, the position of the arch and the volume of the prosthesis may require a careful selection of the abutment shapes. Occasionally, it is easier to resolve such difficulties by recording an impression directly from the fixtures, by removing the healing abutments. (Such problems are more common in the maxillae.) The abutments are then selected in the laboratory when the trial set-up has been verified.

Once the abutments, either definitive or healing, have been placed, the soft tissues can be sutured around them and a pack placed. This is the same type as that used in periodontal surgery and is held in place by special healing caps placed on the abutments. The patient must be advised to avoid undue pressure on this region whilst the soft tissues are healing, and to utilise hot salt water and chlorhexidine mouthwashes.

After about 7–10 days the pack may be taken off, the sutures removed and the denture reinserted. Where healing is not sufficiently completed, this stage may need to be delayed until two weeks after the second-stage surgery. The healing caps should then be replaced to protect the tops of the abutments and prevent debris collect in the fixing holes. This is especially important where implants are opposed by natural teeth as some patients grind these against the TMAs, causing considerable damage. Some implant systems include an additional smaller type of healing cap for use once the pack has been removed.

The dentures will need to be relieved over the healing caps, and this is best achieved as described above. The prosthesis is then modified with a tissue conditioner and returned to the patient. In the case of mandibular implants, the denture is particularly susceptible to fracture. It is often necessary, therefore, to reinforce it either by thickening it with acrylic resin, which can make it unacceptably bulky, or by incorporating a metal stainless-steel strengthener of 1 mm diameter wire below the necks of the anterior teeth. This will provide some resistance against fracture, although wire of this dimension will hold the denture components together if it should break rather than contribute significantly to the strength of the prosthesis.

Recording impressions

The recording of impressions in implant treatment requires great precision as the implants are essentially rigid and incapable of orthodontic movement. Thus inaccuracies will result in a poorly fitting prosthesis and high stresses, both in the superstructure and in the bone around the implant.

The impressions must also record the relationships of the implants to the adjacent soft tissues and functional sulci, so as to aid in visualising the final outcome and assist in the positioning of the teeth and gumwork on the prosthesis.

As most dental implants do not project far above the soft tissues when first exposed, the use of impression copings is essential so as to record accurately the position and orientation of the fixtures. These manufactured devices are usually implant-specific and may be linked to the implant in a variety of ways, of which screwing with an integral threaded component, screwing with a separate screw and a push-fit with a dowel are the most common.

A further subdivision is between tapered copings, which can remain *in situ* when the impression is removed, and those which have an irregularity which necessitates their removal with the impression. These usually suffer from the need to gain access to their fixing screws prior to withdrawing the impression. As a result, it is necessary to have access holes in the top of the tray as well as room in the mouth to use a screwdriver. They do, however, avoid the need to relocate the copings in the impression, which is a potential

source of inaccuracy, and may also be rigidly linked in the mouth prior to recording the overall impression, which can also improve precision.

The tapered coping, on the other hand, is particularly valuable where access is restricted, for example in the more distal sites.

The Brånemark implant system incorporates both types of coping and is the type described in this chapter, although the procedures are equally valid for any other design of a similar generic pattern.

When fabricating a fixed bridge prosthesis in the edentulous jaw it is necessary to record primary impressions for the fabrication of special trays and as an aid in treatment planning. To do this, the healing caps should be removed, and if necessary the tightness of the screws joining the abutments to the fixtures checked, as has been described in Chapter 5. A suitable stock impression tray should then be selected. This must have sufficient depth, and it is usual to employ a box tray so as to clear the copings adequately. As these cannot be removed with the impression, a tapered design should be selected and then placed on the fixtures. A check is then made that the tray can be easily inserted. If not, then a different pattern should be chosen. Plastic disposable impression trays can be very useful in this context as they may be modified by grinding to provide a better fit. This is particularly important if long copings are being used as these can restrict access to the mouth. The tray will usually require modification to ensure an appropriate record of the sulci and the areas between and particularly distal to the implants. This is best achieved with impression compound. Care should be taken to remove the impression before the compound has set, lest it become fixed on the copings; this is more likely to occur if the implants are not parallel. The hole in the compound made by the coping should then be enlarged with a mirror handle to provide clearance for a subsequent wash impression in alginate. Any peripheral deficiencies can be made good by modifying the compound, which should next be chilled, coated with a suitable adhesive and the wash impression made.

As the impressions of the copings in the compound are deep and tend to trap air they should first be filled with a small amount of alginate injected from a disposable syringe to prevent the copings being misplaced in the consequent void.

Once the impression has set it may be removed, rinsed with water, inspected, sprayed with a disinfectant and the copings removed from the implants and placed in the impression, which should then be returned to the laboratory.

It is also desirable at this stage in the treatment to confirm that the abutments are of the correct length. Too short and cleaning will be difficult, too long and there will be inadequate room for the superstructure. Where room is limited, a final decision on this may require the use of a trial denture, which may therefore have to be made before making the final impressions. If healing abutments have been used, then these will be replaced with the definitive components at this stage.

The recording of working impressions is carried out with special trays and an elastomeric impression material. Where the copings are initially to be linked before recording the overall impression, then a medium viscosity addition cured silicone material may be loaded in the tray, combined with a light-bodied wash injected around the implants. Where the copings are to remain *in situ* when the impression is removed, then a stiffer material is more appropriate, such as a polyether.

The impression procedure has three distinct stages: the recording of the sulci, the optional linking of the implants (unless they are to remain *in situ*) and the overall impression.

An impression tray for use with screw-retained copings is shown in **6.24**. They are made in acrylic resin, spaced 1.5 mm from the underlying tissues, and incorporate windows to allow for the removal of the fixing screws. These are blocked temporarily with modelling wax to seal the tray whilst recording the impression, which is then removed to gain access to the screws. The periphery of the tray should be checked in a similar fashion to when recording an impression of an edentulous mouth, and a check made that the margins of the opening are level with the tops of the screws. If they are considerably below the surface of the tray then this should be trimmed so as to prevent them becoming enclosed in the impression, which makes their removal difficult. This problem may be overcome by using long screws, albeit at the cost of some difficulty in inserting the impression tray, particularly where its borders have been modified with compound.

When using a fixed prosthesis, an impression of the sulci should be recorded which extends beyond the planned periphery of the appliance. As fixed superstructures cannot be used with flanges similar to those on a complete denture, due to oral hygiene problems, there is no need to record fully the functional sulcus. Depending on the tray extension and viscosity of the impression material, some operators prefer to modify the periphery with a viscous material such as impression compound or an elastomeric putty. The impression copings should be placed on the abutments prior to this so as to ensure that the modified tray can be inserted and removed over them.

If it is desired to link the copings then this should be done next. The purpose of this is to record precisely the relationship of the fixtures and produce a robust impression which will not distort during pouring. The two most common techniques for linking the copings are either to use plaster or self-curing acrylic resin. The disadvantages of impression plaster are its weakness in thin sections and its tendency to fracture on removal if it has flowed around non-parallel abutments. Self-curing resin, often marketed under the trade name 'Duralay', requires a framework for support whilst it polymerises and care must be taken to minimise its bulk so as to control the effects of polymerisation shrinkage. This may be achieved by using manufactured copings with plastic extensions which can be trimmed until they almost touch when seated in the mouth. Self-curing acrylic resin may then be flowed over the gap to link them without causing significant distortion due to its minimal bulk. An alternative technique is to use a custom-fabricated cast cobalt chromium bar. This needs only to be roughly trimmed, and should be soldered to one of the copings. Its use is shown in **6.30** and it provides a frame to which the copings can be affixed with a thin layer of resin.

The technique of linking copings with a 'cats-cradle' of dental floss over which self-curing acrylic resin is then run is to be condemned as the relaxation of the tension in the floss, combined with the polymerisation shrinkage of the resin, can lead to considerable inaccuracies.

Once the copings have been linked, the screw heads should be covered with a small amount of carding wax if short screws are being utilised. This will facilitate their retrieval from the subsequent impression but is not required with long screws which will protrude through the wax lid when the tray is placed. The light-bodied elastomer is then flowed around the copings, and the tray loaded and seated. Where short screws have been placed, finger pressure should be applied over the wax lid until the screw heads can be felt with the finger tips. The sulci should then be moulded. When the material sets, the wax lid can be removed, the screws undone and the impression removed, rinsed, inspected and sprayed with disinfectant.

Where the copings remain *in situ*, a non-perforated tray may be used and the impression procedure is similar to that employed when recording impressions of prepared natural teeth.

At the end of this stage, the healing caps should be replaced and the impressions returned to the laboratory where abutment replicas will be mounted on the copings and the impressions poured in modified die stone.

Recording jaw relationships

The recording of jaw relationships and the associated prescription of tooth positions is an essential component of the construction of an implant-stabilised fixed prosthesis. It is, however, one which should initially be carried out as part of treatment planning, since the feasibility of constructing a suitable prosthesis must be confirmed prior to implant placement. The subsequent record will therefore be required to verify the earlier version and ensure that the teeth are in the most advantageous positions prior to constructing the cast framework on which they will be placed.

The record is normally made using a conventional acrylic base plate and wax rim. This should fit over the abutments and be extended in a similar fashion to an orthodox base. Whilst it is possible to construct a base incorporating holes over the abutments to which it may be secured with screws, this is not without its problems, as the frequent insertion and removal of the screws is time-consuming and can lead to wear of the threads in the TMAs. An alternative is to secure the base *in situ* only when making the final record of the jaw relationship. Usually, however, the fit of the base around the abutments ensures enough stability to produce an accurate record without resort to such measures.

The jaw registration procedure is essentially similar to that used for a patient who is edentulous in one or both jaws, although particular care must be taken with the positioning of the teeth in view of the need to link them to the underlying implants whilst maintaining room for oral hygiene and controlling occlusal loads.

The final record of the relationship may be made with a wax wafer or a registration paste. The selection of teeth also follows conventional principles, although with a fixed superstructure it should be borne in mind that the teeth will need to obscure the underlying fixtures where possible. This may place constraints on the mould chosen.

The occlusal scheme which it is intended to use will depend on the clinical situation and is not implant-specific, although care should be taken to avoid undue forces on the superstructure. In the edentulous arch, group function should be provided if opposing a natural dentition and balanced articulation if opposing a complete denture. There is some evidence that the use of balanced articulation when the superstructure opposes a natural dentition may reduce the loads on the fixtures. This may not be achievable, but a canine-guided occlusal scheme should be avoided due to the high localised forces which can result. Where the arch is edentulous then the retruded contact and intercuspal positions of the mandible should be coincident, whilst in general, in restoration of the partially edentulous arch, a conformative approach should be used in this respect.

Once the registration has been completed and the rims related to the opposing dentition or record rim at the desired vertical and horizontal relationship, a face bow record should be made so that the casts may be mounted correctly on an articulator. The technician next prepares a trial denture for clinical assessment. It is important that this follows the prescribed degree of lip support, and for a fixed superstructure will thus be of an open-faced design.

An alternative approach to recording the jaw relationship may be adopted after the second operation. This involves duplicating the temporary denture when it is adjusted to fit over the healing caps. This duplicate may then be used to create a replica suitable for registering the jaw relation, as well as a suitable model on which to form a special tray. This should have an anterior open box form sufficient to encompass the impression copings. Using this method, primary casts and classical record rims can be dispensed with.

Once this stage has been completed the healing caps are replaced and the patient discharged.

Trial appliances

Before proceeding to casting the metal superstructure it is essential to have a trial prosthesis made and checked in the mouth. The purposes of this are to ensure that both patient and dentist are satisfied with the appearance which is produced and that the positions of the teeth are satisfactory from the technical viewpoint.

The trial denture usually incorporates a temporary acrylic base, similar to that used for complete dentures, so as to provide the necessary stability. This is readily achieved by ensuring that it fits around the abutments. However, the bulk of the base makes it somewhat difficult to envisage the final result. A more realistic, and fragile, alternative is to have the teeth set on an acrylic base with similar contours to the final prosthesis. This is mounted on the abutments and provides little potential for altering tooth positions.

The technical criteria to be satisfied relate to the relations of the teeth with the opposing dentition and the underlying ridge and implants. It is important to consider the following points:

- Will the teeth in the prosthesis have to be linked to the abutments in such a way as to result in heavy torque on the implants?
- Do the teeth provide an acceptable appearance?
- Is the space below the prosthesis adequate for cleaning purposes?
- Can the mucosal aspect of the prosthesis be made convex or at least flat, so as to aid cleaning? Concave surfaces tend to collect plaque and calculus unless access can be gained with a brush.
- Is there a risk of food stagnation under the appliance?
- Have the anterior teeth been set so far labially as to result in the lip becoming trapped below their labial margins? Can this be prevented with a short flange, and if so can the patient keep it clean?
- Will it be possible to gain access to the fixing screws, if any, for the superstructure with the teeth set in the proposed positions?
- Will the teeth mask the abutments from the front of the mouth? This may be a problem if the implants are not in the same positions as some of the teeth.

It is also a sensible precaution at this stage to verify the accuracy of the master cast before further time is invested in technical and clinical work. This may be done with a check bar made in the laboratory. Where a metal bar has been used to link the copings at the impression stage, this can be readily modified by fixing it to impression copings mounted on the dummy abutments in the master cast. The resultant frame can then be removed and used clinically to confirm the accuracy of the master cast. To do this the copings in the bar should be positioned over the abutments and the fixing screws partly inserted. One screw in turn should then be tightened, the others remaining slack, and the fit of the coping checked by eye. Any visible gaps indicate an unacceptable fit and the need to re-record the master impression. An alternative technique, where a metal bar has not been used, is to employ one made of self-curing acrylic resin which has been made to fit passively on the master cast. These are fixed to the abutments via the gold cylinders which will eventually be incorporated in the cast gold superstructure. The disadvantages of using an acrylic bar for verification are the technical difficulties of overcoming its polymerisation shrinkage and the flexibility of the material.

Whilst there is considerable laboratory research evidence as to the problems which may arise as a result of an ill-fitting superstructure, these have not yet been quantified or assessed clinically. In these circumstances the recommendation is that superstructures with visible deficiencies of fit, when placed passively on the abutments, should not be used.

Once these matters have been dealt with to the clinician's and patient's satisfaction, the healing caps may be replaced and the patient discharged.

The cast framework

The next phase of treatment is for the technician, in consultation with the clinician, to make the metal framework for the prosthesis. A choice between a cast gold alloy beam and a welded and milled titanium framework (Procera technique) exists. The dimensions of the frameworks are little different and it is the authors' impression that more complex welded shapes fit positively without the problems accompanying casting shrinkage, which are not always overcome even when using recommended spruing and casting techniques. It is, however, necessary to have the framework produced in a specialist laboratory.

The first stage of the process involves the production of plaster overcasts (indices) of the trial appliance so that the teeth may be correctly related to the abutment replicas. The gold cylinders are then placed on the abutments and held in position with screws. The amount of vertical space should be carefully checked as it may be necessary to use short cylinders if room is restricted. It will also be apparent if there is a conflict between the position of the teeth and the cylinders. The technician must confirm that: (i) access for the fixing screws in the cylinders is not inhibited, (ii) the teeth do not overlap the abutments, (iii) there will be room for the framework between the cylinders and the teeth. On occasion a decision must be made to reposition some of them.

The framework is then developed using the acrylic resin bar, if employed earlier, as a base on which to evolve the casting. The design of the cantilever beam is completed by deciding on the shape of the beam, the method of retaining the teeth (e.g. posts, tagging, beading) and which parts will form part of the polished surface contours not to be covered by acrylic resin. It is accepted that some designs are now executed in porcelain bonded to a suitable precious alloy but this technique will be referred to in Chapter 7 for its use in partial prostheses.

Important factors to be born in mind when waxing up the bar are:

- **Oral hygiene.** It is important to produce a shape which facilitates oral hygiene, and the technician should have available a range of hygiene aids to ensure that the shape which he is producing is one which can be cleaned by the patient. Allowance must, of course, be made for the more restricted access in the mouth compared with the bench top. The mucosal surface of the casting should preferably be flat, or slightly convex if cleaning has to be by means of floss as this cannot reach a concavity. Interproximally it is often necessary to use a small 'bottle brush', and this should be checked against the wax-up, making allowance for the teeth, which will reduce access.
- **Tooth retention.** The framework should incorporate adequate retention tags and, where necessary, metal backings to protect the teeth. These inevitably create difficulties in producing a natural appearance and whilst they can protect the teeth they indicate also that heavy loads may fall upon the prosthesis. Such eventualities should be considered at the treatment planning stage. Where occlusal loads on the prosthesis are thought to be likely to be excessive then either an alternative form of treatment should be contemplated or implant numbers, dimensions and locations planned so as to maximise their collective load-carrying capability.
- **Occlusion.** This should be designed to minimise high localized loads on the super-structure. Balanced articulation or group function are preferred. Canine guidance should be avoided.
- **Occlusal material.** Many workers recommend the use of acrylic occlusal surfaces on implant-stabilised bridges so as to minimise occlusal loads through their 'cushioning' effect. There is no clinical research evidence to support this contention, and porcelain teeth are more wear-resistant. Unfortunately, they are not always readily joined on to the casting, and acrylic teeth are more flexible in this respect. If high quality, heavily cross-linked acrylic teeth are used then wear is less of a problem. Manufacturers are also introducing modified acrylic teeth which are suitable for implant prosthesis and claimed to be highly wear resistant.Consideration may be given to the use of metal occlusal surfaces. However, in general it is undesirable to use materials with different wear characteristics on one occlusal surface unless this can be regularly monitored. There is some evidence that where distal cantilevers on implant-stabilised bridges are slightly out of occlusion then the loads on them are significantly reduced. Such sensitivity to occlusal contours indicates that differential wear could produce high local stresses.
- **Strength.** The superstructure should be waxed-up so as to have adequate strength. In general this requires a cross-section of 8×5 mm and distal cantilevers no longer than 13 mm in the lower jaw and 10 mm in the upper, using a Type IV gold alloy. Similar constrains may apply to the welded titanium framework. It should, however, be remembered that accurate data on these points are not available due to the considerable variation in patients' anatomies, and the clinician should therefore tend towards caution.
- **Screw access.** It must be remembered that the clinician will require easy access to the screws which hold the prosthesis in place. This will often be through the occlusal surface of the teeth, and whilst it is a factor decided at the treatment planning stage and later when the implants are inserted the technician can aid screw manipulation by shaping the guide holes appropriately. This is particularly important where the screws are well below the occlusal plane and the implants less advantageously angled. In these circumstances the holes through the superstructure should provide precise guidance for the screwdriver.

There is considerable research evidence of the strains which can arise as a result of using ill-fitting superstructures, and it is thought that these can lead to loss of integration and fracture of implant components and sometimes the superstructure itself. Unfortunately, these matters have not yet been quantified, nor is there a method available for measuring clinically the deficiency of fit of a superstructure other than visual estimation. In these circumstances, castings should be regarded as unsatisfactory if marginal deficiencies can be seen with the naked eye, or the casting fails to remain in place on all abutments when an individual gold cylinder is tightened. If there is a similar error on the master cast, the framework should either be sectioned and resoldered at the site of the error, or be remade. Where there are several faults such that none of the gold cylinders fit then the latter course is to be preferred. Such problems are less common if a welded titanium superstructure is used. When the problem lies in an inadequate master cast then the working impression should be retaken prior to fabricating a new casting.

Errors in the jaw relationship are uncommon when satisfactory stable jaw relations have existed with the previous dentures. Should there be any minor occlusal errors detected at this stage then a registration of the occlusion may conveniently be made on the framework. If this has enough contacts with the opposing dentition, either artificial or natural, then this may be achieved with a thin layer of registration paste on the contact areas. Where the casting lacks adequate numbers of contacts then it should first be built up with hard wax in the relevant sites so as to create a platform on which the registration may be made with paste.

Trial stage

Before proceeding to completion of the bridge prosthesis it is essential to check the framework with the teeth waxed-up, as subsequent alterations are time-consuming and costly. This will provide both clinician and patient with a final opportunity to confirm that they are both satisfied with the appliance from the technical and aesthetic viewpoints. The framework should be screwed into position and then the appearance checked from all directions whilst the patient relaxes, and also speaks and moves the lips as extensively as is compatible with normal activity. It is at this stage that minor changes in the positions of the teeth, level of gingival margins and extension of the flanges are often required. It is also important to check for access for oral hygiene.

At this time it is essential to examine the surface contours of the prosthesis so that no obstruction occurs to movements of the lips or tongue during speaking and swallowing.

When treating a patient with only a mandibular implant-stabilised prosthesis, for whom new conventional dentures have been previously constructed, it is assumed that the maxillary one will be fully retentive and stable. Hence the centric and eccentric occlusions should exhibit balance and the mandibular trial fixed prosthesis should not destabilise the maxillary denture.

The appliance may then be returned to the laboratory for processing.

Insertion

If all the previous stages have been carried out correctly then this is usually a straightforward procedure. The screw holes in the abutments, if an implant system of that type is being employed, should be checked for obstructions and the prosthesis then screwed into position. It is important when doing this not to trap the cheek inadvertently, as it may collapse in on the appliance, and to tighten the screws sequentially. Initially, they should be tightened only lightly to ensure that the casting is optimally centred over the abutments, and then fully torqued. Before the final tightening a check should be made of the fit of the framework, although it is very unusual for this to have become deficient by this stage.

Before the completed fixed prosthesis is finally screwed into position, it is usual to check the security of the abutments and to record long cone dental X-rays using a parallelling technique in order to confirm the level of the investing bone and the integrity of contact with each fixture. These films produce a reference for subsequent monitoring.

The occlusion and articulation with the appliance in place should next be examined. This may be conveniently done with thin articulating paper followed by adjustment of the occlusal surfaces at the chair side. Where more extensive modification may be required a pre-occlusal registration should be made and the appliance returned to the laboratory for adjustment.

A common problem during the fitting of implant components is the handling of the various tools and small components which can easily be dropped by the gloved hand. Screwdrivers should have a length of dental floss threaded through the handle and tied in a loop which can be passed round the operator's wrist. Screws present more of a challenge, and those with hexagonal sockets are more readily stabilised on the end of a screwdriver whilst being inserted. A small piece of carding wax provides a convenient method of relating the two and, indeed, a short length of this material provides an effective screw holder for starting a screw in a difficult location. Alternatively, a piece of electrical heat-shrinkable sleeving can be effective in keeping a screw in place on a screwdriver where access to the fixture is awkward.

Once the screws have been tightened, the holes through which they are inserted are sealed temporarily with a small amount of silicone impression material injected through a fine syringe. This forms an effective, rapidly removed, seal which also provides an additional and convenient record of the type of screw head in use; something not always evident if the hole is very deep and angled unfavourably.

The patient must now be given thorough instruction in oral hygiene procedures. A wide range of aids is available, consisting basically of flosses of various types, small bottle brushes, and interspace brushes. Patients often find that, for reasons of personal preference, local anatomy, manual skills or superstructure design one type of aid is particularly suitable and they should therefore have the opportunity of using a range. **6.62–6.67** illustrate some of these, and it is essential that patients do not leave until they are confident that they can keep their appliance clean.

Maintenance

The patient should be seen for a review appointment after one week and a check made on any problems encountered, followed by a careful examination of the prosthesis and surrounding tissues.

Common problems are:

- **Difficulty with oral hygiene.** The lingual aspects of the mandibular abutments are often particularly troublesome. This may not be evident to the patient and will require reinforcement by the dentist or hygienist. Some patients find the procedures difficult to master and should be encouraged to demonstrate these in the surgery. The patient may require several training sessions with a hygienist who should confirm that the mucosal cuffs are not tender, inhibiting proper cleaning. Also, the patient should be encouraged to close the mouth partially so that the lips can be pulled down and away from the prosthesis. Many patients need to be encouraged to wear spectacles to inspect the results of their cleaning.
- **Food collection under the prosthesis.** There is little that can usually be done to overcome this problem, which tends to reduce with time as the necessary oral gymnastic skills develop. Sometimes patients find a small obturator helpful, as described below.
- **Speech problems.** These usually arise as a result of the gap between the superstructure and the underlying tissues, and are more common with maxillary appliances. Such problems tend to decrease with time, and can sometimes be helped with a small acrylic or soft rubber obturator or bung. Some patients find the cure worse than the problem!

- **Looseness of an opposing denture.** This is particularly common where an implant-stabilised mandibular prosthesis opposes an upper complete denture. Previously the patient may have been content with the performance of the maxillary prosthesis, but now finds it relatively loose. Patients should always be warned of this possibility, which is difficult to overcome if a soundly designed and fabricated upper denture has been fitted. In some cases, recourse to a maxillary implant-stabilised appliance may be needed, although unfortunately this may not be practicable and should, in any case, have been considered during treatment planning.
- **Cheek biting.** This is usually related to the position of the upper and lower teeth, and often associated with inadequate buccal overlap of the upper teeth in relation to the lower ones. If that is the case then judicious grinding of the teeth so as to round the angle between the occlusal and buccal surfaces and move the buccal cusps of the lower teeth lingually can produce an improvement. In other situations it is caused by problems of adaptability, especially in patients who may have been unable to use a conventional lower prosthesis–thus giving their cheeks and tongue free reign in the oral cavity.
- Other problems are sometimes encountered and are described in Chapter 9.

Once the patient and dentist are satisfied with the performance of the appliance the patient may be discharged for a longer period. Before doing so, the holes over the screws should be sealed with a base layer of silicone rubber capped with a composite filling material. There is no need to seal shallow holes in metal frameworks.

SUMMARY OF THE STAGES IN THE CONSTRUCTION OF A FIXED BRIDGE PROSTHESIS

Some of these phases are laboratory based. More than one phase may occur at a clinical visit, for example, recording jaw relationships and confirming the accuracy of the master cast (Phases 8 and 9).

Phase 1: Record primary impressions

- Recorded over healing abutments or after exchange with permanent abutments.

Phase 2: Position permanent abutments

- Remove healing abutment from healed cuff.
- Measure depth to fixture head.
- Select permanent abutment in order to project surface at least 2 mm above the cuff. Exact dimension dependent on vertical space available.
- Locate abutment as appropriate for design.
- Place healing caps on abutments.

Phase 3: Design special trays

- Ensure correct coverage.
- Provide access for impression transfer copings.
- If preferred, design cast bar for impression procedure.

Phase 4: Record master impressions

- Remove healing caps.
- Attach impression transfer copings with long or short fixing screws.
- Insert special tray, check fit and extension with sufficient clearance for copings.
- Modify tray periphery with impression material if required.
- Apply adhesive, record elastomeric impression with correct border moulding procedure.
- If using impression bar, then locate this with self-curing resin and then record impression.
- Remove impression and replace healing caps.

Phase 5: Pour master casts

- Screw brass replica abutments to transfer copings.
- Box and pour impression in modified dental stone.

Phase 6: Construct check bar

Phase 7: Design record blocks

- Outline base, wax-out undercuts on cast.
- Prepare light or self-cured acrylic resin base with access for fixing screws.
- Add wax rim.

Phase 8: Record jaw relations (including transfer face bow record)

- Select teeth.

Phase 9: Confirm accuracy of master cast with check bar

Phase 10: Construct trial appliance

Phase 11: Trial insertion

- Confirm jaw relations after removing healing caps.
- Examine facial support offered by arch.
- Confirm positions of artificial teeth. In particular, check the necks of the teeth during maximum lip activity.

Phase 12: Prepare the cast framework

- Index the try-in on the master cast.
- Position appropriate gold cylinders with fixing screws on brass replicas.
- Check clearance with teeth using the index.
- Wax-up bar to provide support for teeth, and adequate space for cleaning of abutments and superstructure.
- Invest and solder the bar to the cylinders.

Phase 13: Try-in the framework

- Confirm each cylinder has a passive, exact fit upon the titanium implant.
- If necessary, make registration check record using registration paste.

Phase 14: Prepare bridge for finishing

- Replace waxed-up prosthesis on master cast.
- Place long screws through gold cylinders into replica abutments.
- Invest mounted prosthesis in dental plaster.
- Boil out wax, pack flask with heat-curing resin and process.
- Remove from flask.
- Replace prosthesis and master cast on articulator. Check occlusion.

Phase 15: Insert completed prosthesis

- Remove healing caps, check abutment screws if employed in design being used.

- Insert bridge and record check record to remount case. Refine occlusal balance.
- Reinsert bridge.

Phase 16: Record long cone X-rays to show marginal bone level

Phase 17: Reassess prosthesis

- Examine components including security of the gold screws.
- Monitor oral hygiene standard.

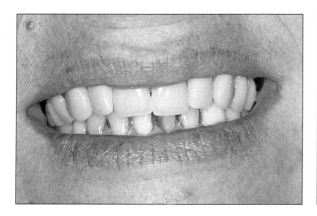

6.1 This patient has an edentulous maxilla and a restored dentate lower arch. She is to be treated with an implant-stabilised fixed prosthesis in the upper jaw. The trial denture, shown here, provides a pleasing appearance and confirms the feasibility of implant treatment.

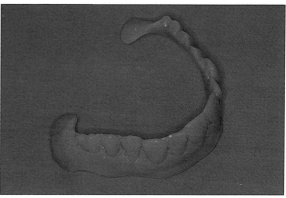

6.2 A surgeon's guide or template has been made from the trial denture using self-curing acrylic resin. This indicates the positions of the teeth on the final prosthesis.

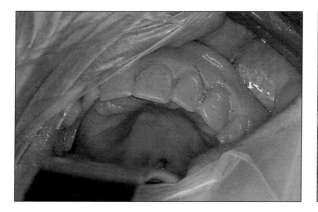

6.3 The guide is used at surgery to assist in the correct placing of the implants.

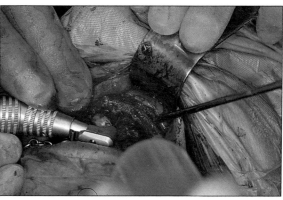

6.4 A pilot hole is drilled in the bone.

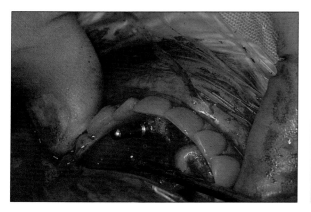

6.5 A guide pin has been inserted in the projected implant site to confirm the position and orientation of the hole.

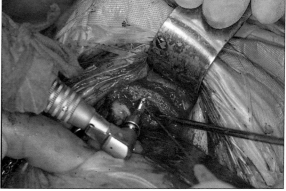

6.6 After preparation of the cavity in the bone, an implant is inserted with a mechanical driver rotating at slow speed to minimise thermal trauma to the bone.

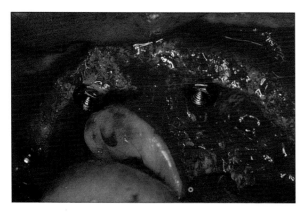

6.7 Implants have been inserted in the anterior part of the maxillae.

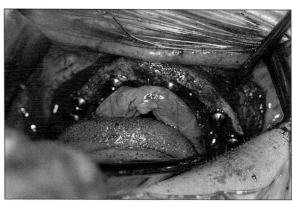

6.8 Cover screws are then placed over the implants to prevent ingrowth of bone into the screw holes in the fixtures, and the wound closed.

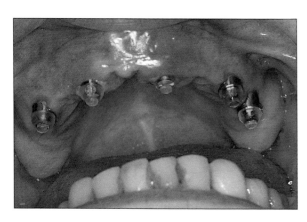

6.9 Two weeks after the second-stage surgery the patient is ready for the prosthetic phase of treatment.

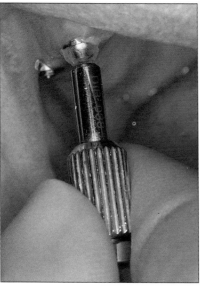

6.10 The healing caps are removed with a socket screwdriver.

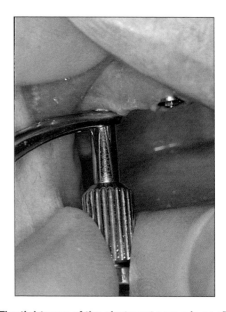

6.11 The tightness of the abutment screw is confirmed. The forceps applied to the abutment prevent a torque being applied to the fixture. More effective tightening is achieved in the Brånemark system using an electronically controlled mechanical driver rather than the finger-held screwdriver shown here (see 3.50).

6.12 Tapered impression copings may be used for recording primary impressions. A coping is shown here with a replica implant abutment which is used in the laboratory.

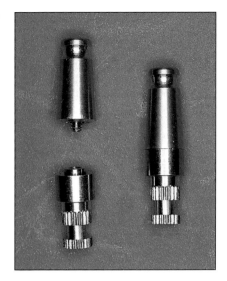

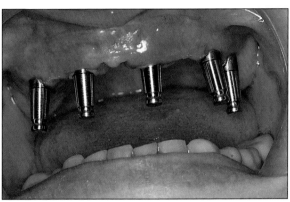

6.13 The impression copings have been screwed onto the abutments.

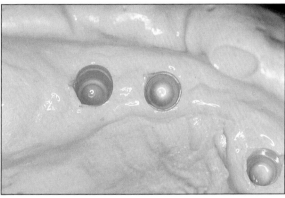

6.14 A primary impression is recorded in alginate (irreversible hydrocolloid). Note the record of the groove in the copings which ensures their correct repositioning in the impression.

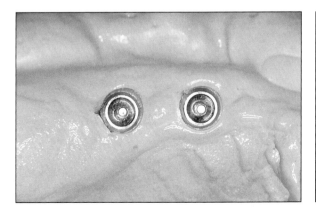

6.15 The impression copings have been replaced in the impression.

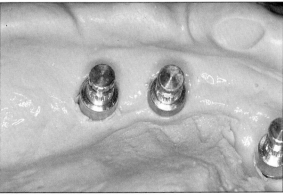

6.16 Impression copings and replica abutments mounted in the impression.

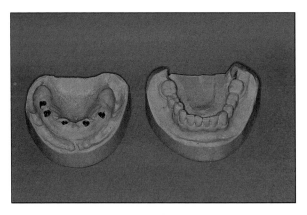

6.17 The primary casts are then poured and trimmed.

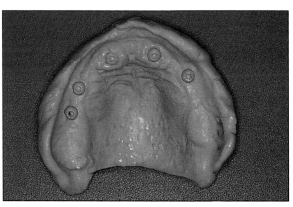

6.18 A thin mix of alginate, used without an adhesive, provides a convenient disclosing medium for adjusting the denture.

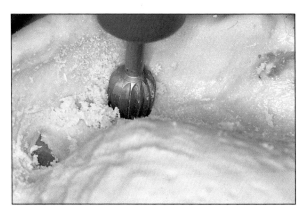

6.19 The denture is then relieved at the sites of the healing caps.

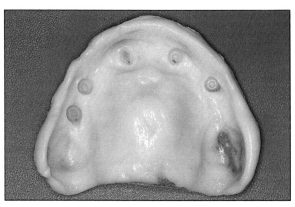

6.20 A tissue-conditioning material is next placed in the denture to improve its stability and minimise soft-tissue trauma.

Working impressions

6.21 The square impression coping, shown here together with its screw and a standard replica abutment, may be used for recording second impressions.

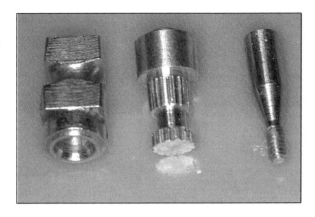

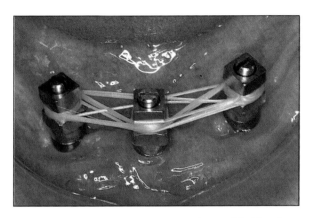

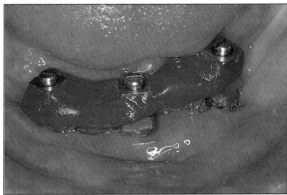

6.22, 6.23 The once popular technique of linking impression copings intra-orally using dental floss and self-curing acrylic resin is prone to distortion.

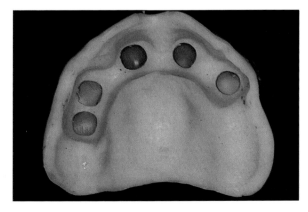

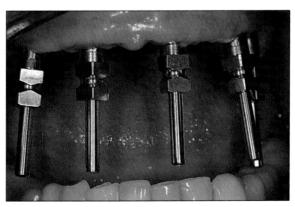

6.24 Where screw-retained impression copings are used it is necessary to place access holes in the impression tray. These are covered with a wax lid to prevent escape of impression material.

6.25 An impression may be recorded in a stiff elastomeric material without linking the copings. Long screws make it easier to release the copings when the impression material has set. Where the gape is limited or there are opposing teeth, it is usually impossible to insert the impression tray.

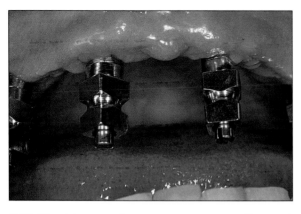

6.26 Short impression screws are normally used with this type of coping.

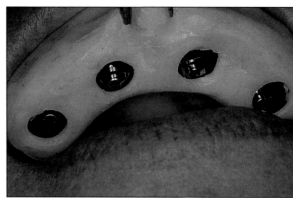

6.27 The impression tray should be checked to ensure that there is adequate access for releasing the impression coping screws.

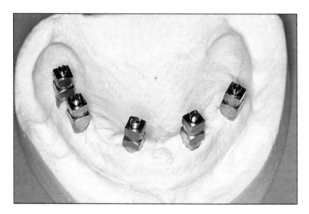

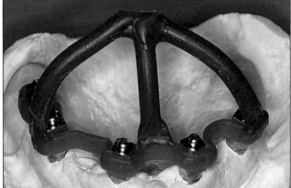

6.28, 6.29 An alternative method of linking impression copings is to use a custom-fabricated cast cobalt chromium bar. This is shown waxed-up on the primary cast.

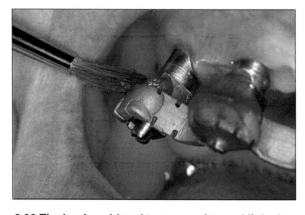

6.30 The bar is soldered to one coping and linked to the others using self-curing acrylic resin. The heads of the screws must be coated with wax to prevent the resin locking them in place.

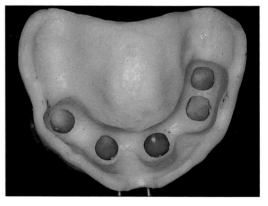

6.31 The impression tray may be border moulded and is then coated with a suitable impression adhesive. The holes, which have been covered with a wax lid, will provide access to the impression coping screws.

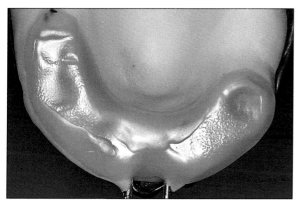

6.32 The wax lid covering the screw access holes.

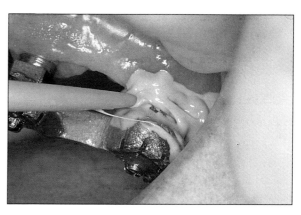

6.33 A low viscosity impression material is then injected around the abutment copings, the impression tray loaded with a medium viscosity material and then seated in the mouth.

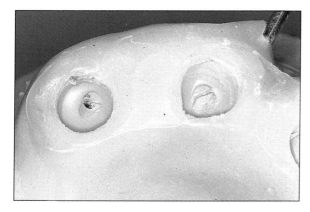

6.34 Once the impression material has set the wax lid can be removed, giving access to the screws, which are then undone to release the impression.

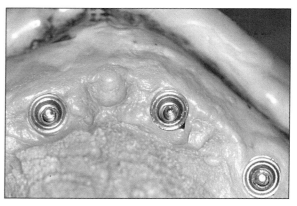

6.35 The fitting surface of the impression showing the impression copings in place.

6.36 Replica abutments are then mounted on the impression copings.

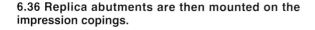

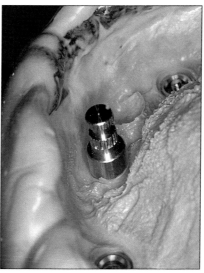

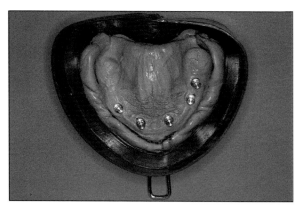

6.37 The impression is next boxed and poured.

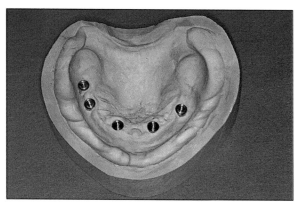

6.38 The master upper cast.

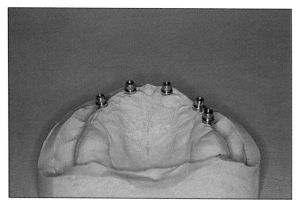

6.39 Gold cylinders are then placed on the abutment replicas.

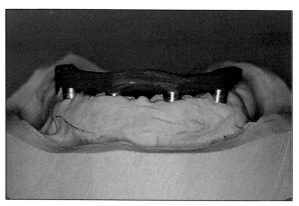

6.40 An acrylic resin check bar is constructed. This links the gold cylinders which should fit passively on the abutments.

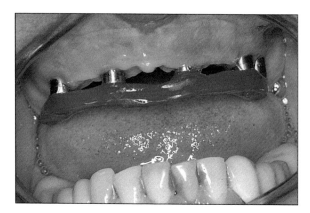

6.41 The check bar is used in the mouth to confirm the accuracy of the master cast.

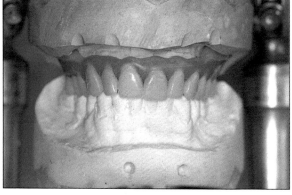

6.42 Following the recording of jaw relationships, the original trial denture is waxed-up to the new master cast.

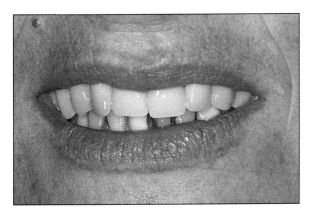

6.43 The trial denture is once again checked in the mouth to confirm the correctness of the tooth positions.

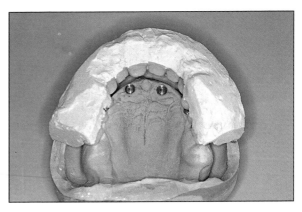

6.44 An overcast is poured in the laboratory to provide an accurate record of the tooth positions.

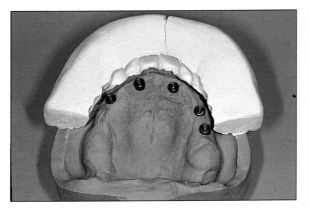

6.45 The overcast is sectioned and used when waxing-up the framework for the implant superstructure. The acrylic check record serves as a base for this.

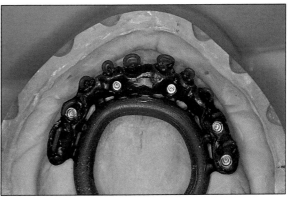

6.46 The waxed-up framework with heavy sprues.

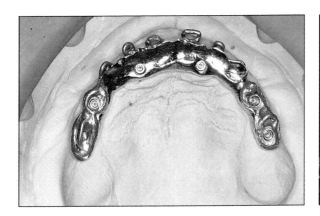

6.47 The completed casting.

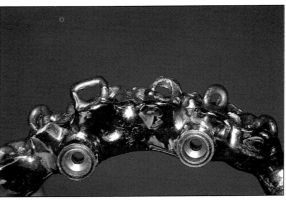

6.48 The mucosal surface of the casting.

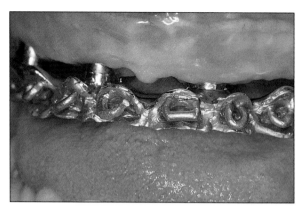

6.49 The casting is then checked in the mouth to confirm the accuracy of its fit.

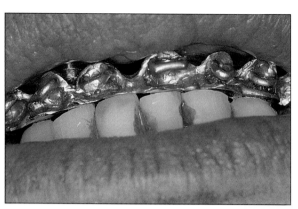

6.50 It is also important to confirm that the occlusal registration is correct.

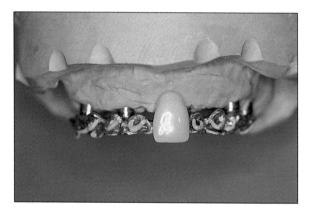

6.51 Using the overcasts the teeth are then waxed-up in position on the framework.

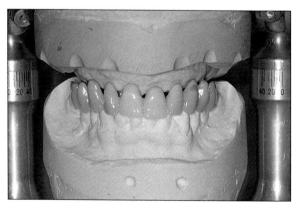

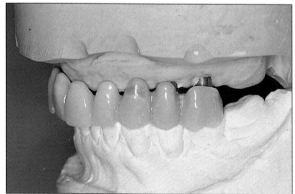

6.52, 6.53 The completed prosthesis.

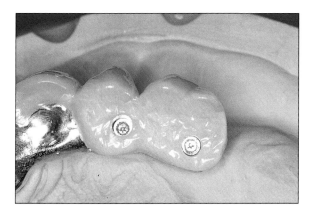

6.54 It is usually necessary to position the artificial teeth buccal to the ridge to provide an appropriate occlusion.

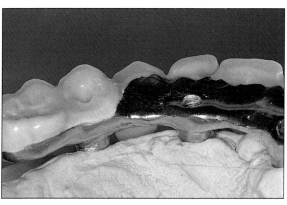

6.55 The fixed prosthesis may be cantilevered distally. It is important to ensure that there is adequate space for oral hygiene.

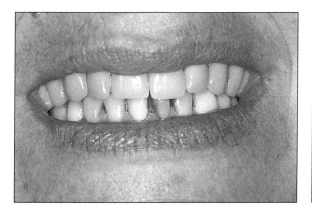

6.56 The prosthesis is then inserted and the occlusion checked and adjusted as necessary.

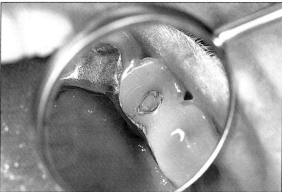

6.57 Access holes to abutment screws may be temporarily filled with a light-bodied elastomeric impression material.

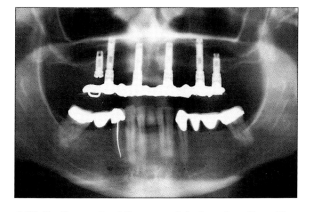

6.58 Radiograph of the completed restoration. The fixture in the 15 region has not been exposed, having been placed as a 'sleeper' for possible use if the adjacent fixture failed.

Review

6.59 The implant superstructure appears to be satisfactory at a review appointment four years after placement.

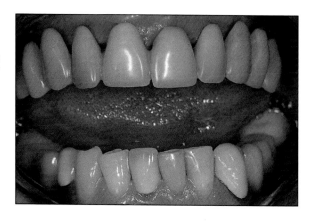

6.60 The superstructure has been removed and demonstrates the high level of oral hygiene which the patient has been able to maintain.

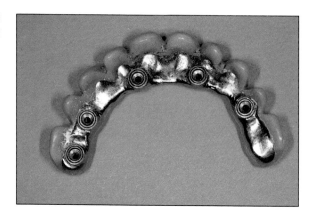

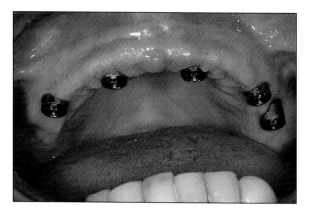

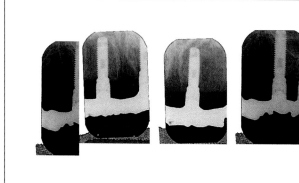

6.61 The tissues around the implants continue to be healthy.

Oral hygiene

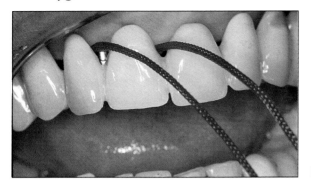
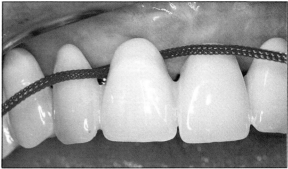

6.62, 6.63 It is essential that the patient receives comprehensive instructions in oral hygiene. This special floss can be looped around the posts and used to clean all their surfaces.

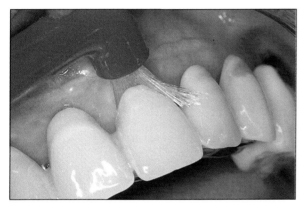

6.64 An interspace brush is a useful aid to cleaning behind ridge-lapped teeth.

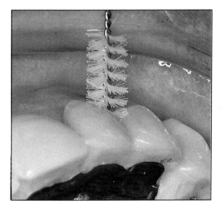

6.65 A miniature bottle brush is useful for cleaning below the superstructure.

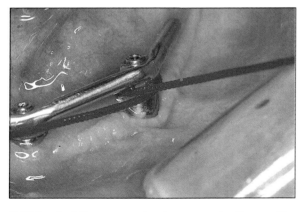

6.66 Implant floss may also be conveniently used to clean abutments employed with overdenture stabilising bars.

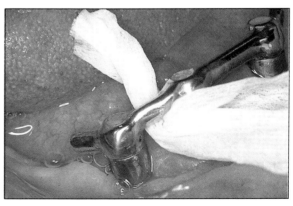

6.67 Dental napkins are another useful hygiene aid.

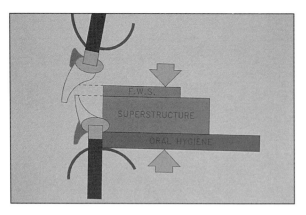

6.68 The superstructure design must provide room for the freeway space and the prosthesis as well as space for hygiene.

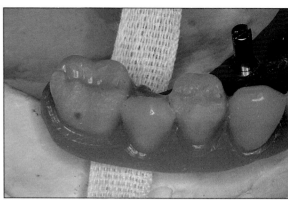

6.69 It is important that the design of the superstructure incorporates provision for hygiene at the construction stage. Here an implant cleaning aid is being used in the laboratory to confirm that adequate space exists below the superstructure.

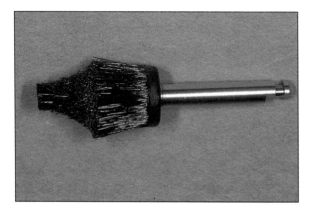

6.70 A range of specially shaped polishing cups and brushes is now available to assist in cleaning implant superstructures and abutments.

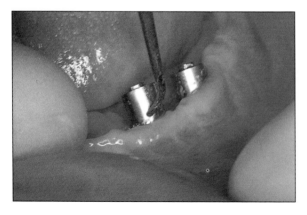

6.71 Some patients are prone to the accumulation of plaque and calculus on their abutments. Hard plastic scalers are available which effectively remove these deposits without causing excessive abrasion of the abutment surface.

Use of healing abutments

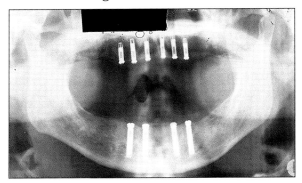

6.72 This patient is being treated with implants in both jaws.

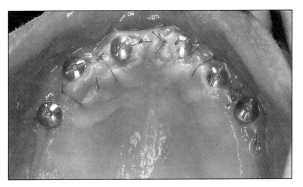

6.73 Healing abutments were placed in the maxillae at the second stage of surgery.

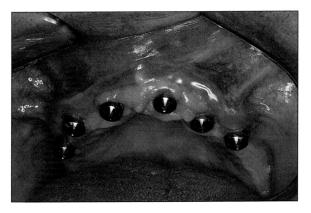

6.74 Two weeks after the second surgical stage the patient is ready for the placing of the more permanent abutments.

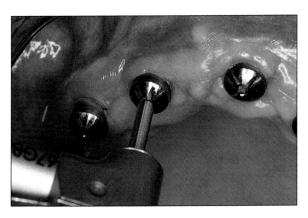

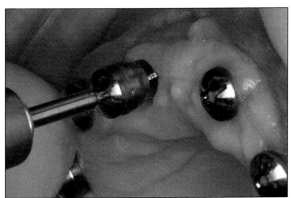

6.75, 6.76 The healing abutments are removed with a mechanical screwdriver.

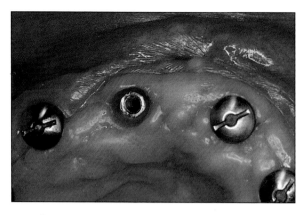

6.77 Once the abutment has been removed, the top of the fixture and the soft-tissue cuff can be seen.

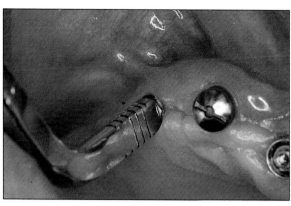

6.78 A graduated probe is used to determine the optimum abutment length.

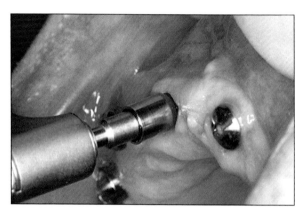

6.79 The abutment is then screwed into position using a mechanical driver.

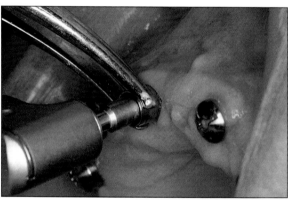

6.80 Once the abutment has been correctly seated on the face of the fixture, the abutment screw is tightened using the forceps to prevent torquing of the fixture.

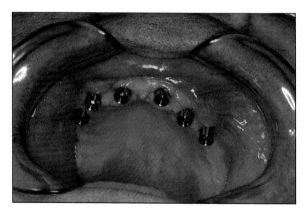

6.81 The abutments in place.

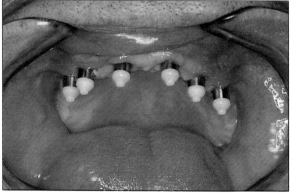

6.82 Healing caps are then placed on the abutments and the patient's temporary denture modified to clear them.

Alternative approaches

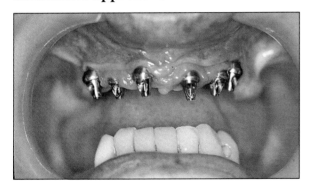

6.83 Angulated abutments used to resolve the difference in alignment of the arch with the position of the fixtures with a Class 2 ii malocclusion.

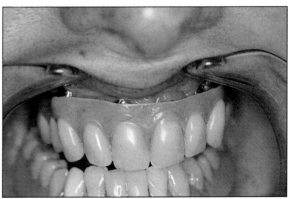

6.84 Flange of the prosthesis spaced from the mucosa and covering the abutments. Necessary because of the high smile line.

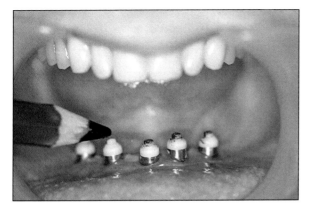

6.85 Healing caps added to the standard abutments and marked with a copying pencil.

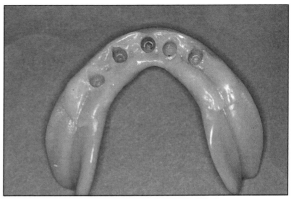

6.86 Temporary lining penetrated in order to accommodate each healing cap and abutment.

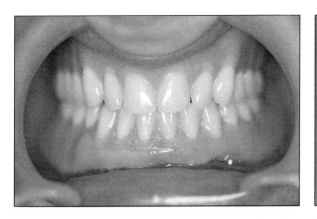

6.87 Complete denture reseated following healing after the operation to connect the abutments.

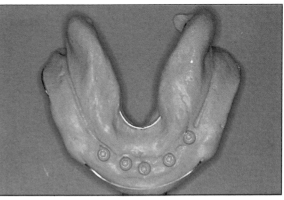

6.88 Primary impression recorded to prepare a special tray.

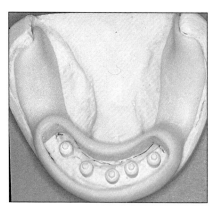

6.89 Open-top box tray prepared for master impression.

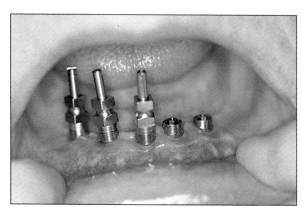

6.90 Attaching impression transfer copings to the abutments.

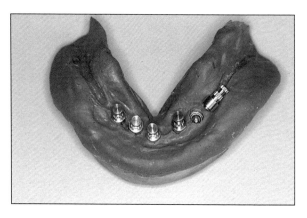

6.91 Completed impression with analogues added.

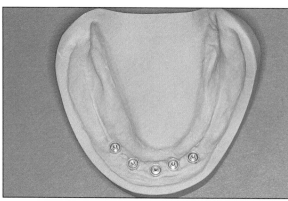

6.92 Master cast incorporating dummy abutments (brass analogues).

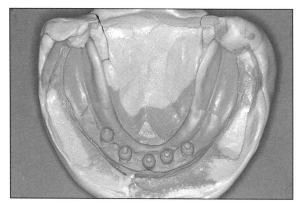

6.93 The use of a copy technique to produce a replica denture which substitutes for the conventional occlusion rim.

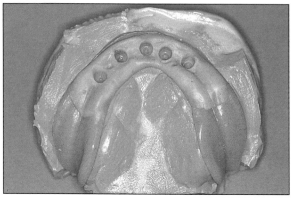

6.94 Silicone putty mould (reverse half).

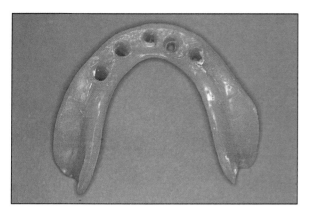

6.95 The wax duplicate pour.

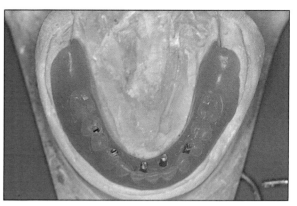

6.96 Duplicate in place on the master cast.

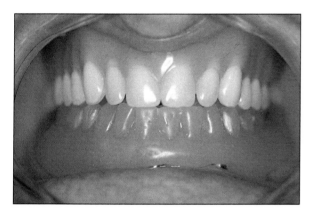

6.97 Recording the jaw relationship.

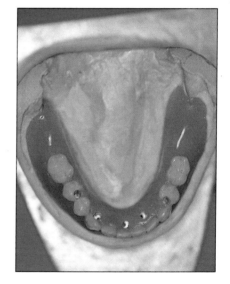

6.98 Artificial resin teeth set up for the trial stage.

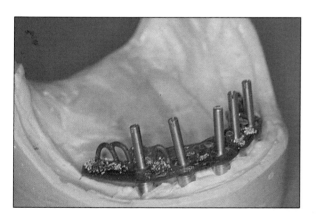

6.99 Wax pattern prepared for the frame of the prosthesis.

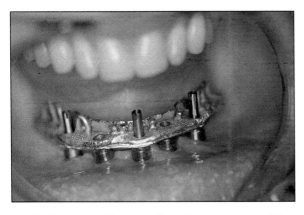

6.100 Frame tried in to confirm the exactness of fit.

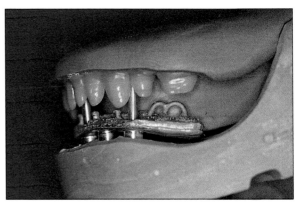

6.101 Setting up the teeth upon the frame using a silicone putty index.

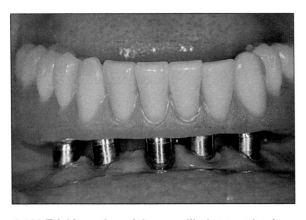

6.102 Trial insertion of the mandibular prosthesis.

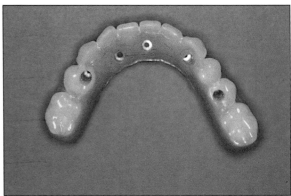

6.103 Divested fixed prosthesis showing the access holes for the fixing screws.

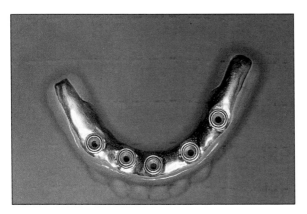

6.104 Convex undersurface of the completed prosthesis.

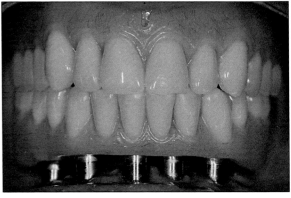

6.105 Completed prosthesis *in situ*.

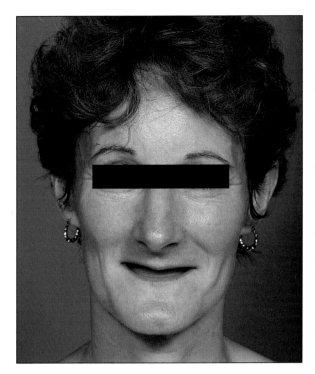
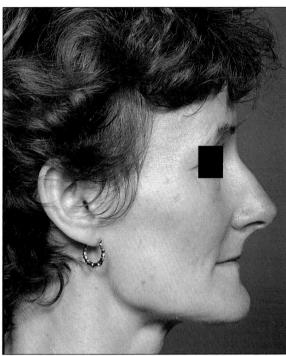

6.106 Patient without complete dentures exhibiting typical appearance.

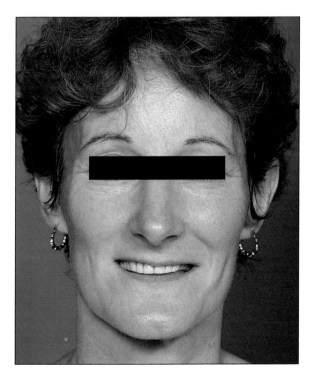

6.107 Patient with old set of complete dentures.

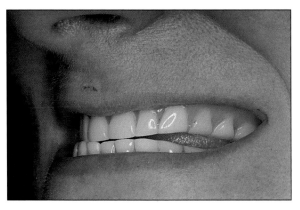

6.108 Dentures exhibiting severe tooth wear after eight years.

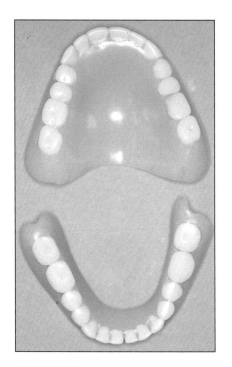

6.109 Old dentures.

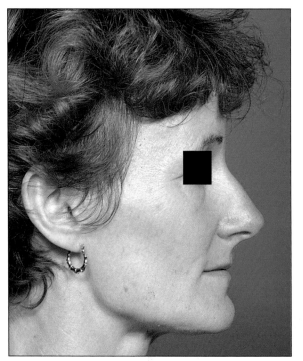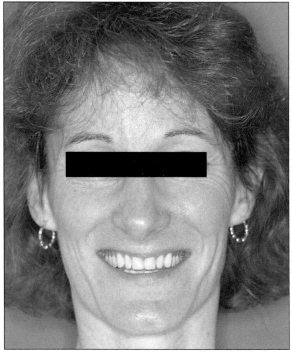

6.110 Patient wearing new upper complete denture and fixed mandibular prosthesis in repose and smiling.

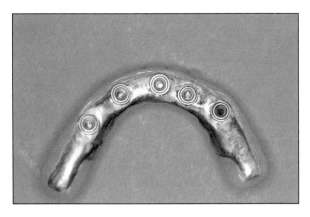

6.111 Mandibular fixed prosthesis.

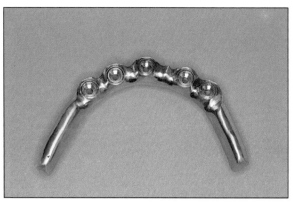

6.112 A welded titanium metal frame produced by the Procera technique.

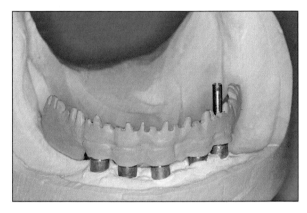

6.113 The frame coated with opaque layer. A single fixing screw demonstrates a passive fit between the frame and each abutment analogue.

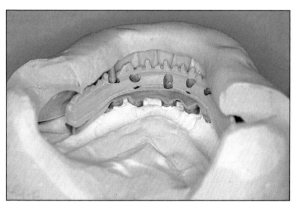

6.114 Index demonstrating the relation of individual retaining posts to the positions of the teeth.

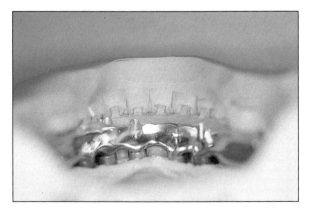

6.115 Close-up view identifying the careful tooth preparation necessary to ensure mechanical retention without excessive loss of the acrylic resin core. Over preparation will produce loss of tooth colour and poor retention on the post.

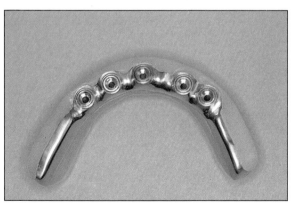

6.116 Inferior surface of the completed prosthesis.

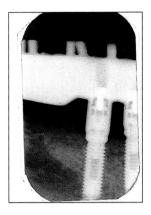 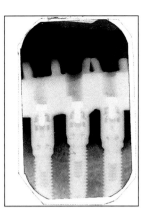

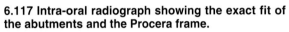

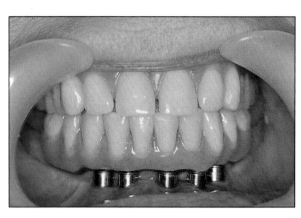

6.117 Intra-oral radiograph showing the exact fit of the abutments and the Procera frame.

6.118 Case showing complete mandibular fixed cantilever prosthesis opposing a maxillary denture.

7. The Partially Edentulous Patient

Introduction

Spaces, or potential spaces, in a dental arch create frequently faced restorative problems, arising as a result of caries, periodontal disease, trauma or hypodontia. These range from the single missing tooth to extensive or irregular tooth loss. The many unfortunate potential effects of untreated tooth loss and the various methods of treating them are well recognised. Among these techniques are treatment with removable partial dentures, adhesive-bonded bridgework, conventional bridgework and orthodontic tooth movement or transplantation to fill a gap in the arch. Whilst a simple partial denture is suitable for immediate tooth replacement, the conventional long-term treatment of a well-preserved dentition is by bridgework. For young persons before the age of maturity, acid etch resin-bonded bridges have been considered appropriate. Unrestored healthy abutment teeth require minimum preparation of enamel surfaces without risk of recurrent caries, except where one retainer has become de-cemented and this has passed unnoticed. Resin-bonded bridges with single pontics exhibit the best outcome, having relatively low construction costs. There is evidence in some studies of de-bonding and the need for re-cementation in 30% of cases. Such treatment is appropriate where the prospect of trauma to conventional bridgework and the liability to damage of the pulps of abutment teeth risk further tooth loss. An estimate of the longevity of conventional bridges is 10 years, with some studies indicating lower survival rates. Neither form of bridgework, however, encourages preservation of the edentulous jaw ridge.

Whilst dental implants were originally developed with the totally edentulous patient in mind, the versatility of modern systems has made their use possible in some partially edentulous patients. They are particularly useful where other methods of restoring the arch are impracticable or could produce an indifferent or uncertain outcome. Dental implants have two major advantages over the alternative methods of tooth replacement: namely, the conservation of alveolar bone in the extraction site and the avoidance of cover or preparation of other dental tissues in the arch.

There are a number of considerations which may make the selection of an implant-stabilised fixed prosthesis in a partially edentulous patient less suitable than a bridge or denture.

- It is relatively more costly to provide this treatment due to the purchase of precision-made components.
- The duration of treatment is longer due to the period required for osseointegration of the implant fixture.
- It is inappropriate where resorption, under-development or trauma has created insufficient bone in the alveolar ridge.
- Sufficient space must exist between suitably aligned adjacent teeth for the fixture, abutment and crown or crowns.
- Inadequate vertical space may exist due to malocclusion or over-eruption of the opposing teeth.
- It may be inappropriate to place a single tooth prosthesis when the remaining dentition exhibits uncontrolled disease or is excessively restored.

The following local considerations should be borne in mind when contemplating possible implant treatment:

- Does the space need to be restored?
- If yes, then what are the alternative methods of restoring the dental arch?
- Could an implant-stabilised prosthesis, including a single crown, give the best result?
- Is it possible to insert the necessary implants into bone of adequate quantity and quality?
- Is it possible to insert the implants in the required positions?
- Could the prosthetic components be correctly sited, bearing in mind tooth relationships in lateral excursions of the mandible?
- What is the prognosis of the remaining teeth? If they were lost would the restoration of the mouth be straightforward or would the fixtures compromise further treatment?
- Would it be necessary to use a tooth- and implant-stabilised bridge? If so what tooth preparation would be required and what would be its prognosis?

Whilst these considerations refer to the implant-stabilised fixed prosthesis, they are also applicable to the single tooth replacement, the special aspects of which are considered later in this chapter.

The answers to some of these questions can be obtained only by preparing diagnostic casts and mounting them on a suitable articulator so that tooth and tooth/ridge relationships can be studied. If there is room to restore the dentition with implants then the necessary radiographic assessments can be made (**7.1, 7.2**). The views selected will depend on the site and the clinical findings. Where space to house the implants within the ridge is limited then tomograms will often be required. The type chosen will depend upon local facilities. However, computerised systems can provide very detailed information in the areas of most importance. Where technically permissible, metal markers should be placed in the trial appliance at the desired sites of the fixtures. These then serve as a guide when assessing the amount of bone available (**7.2**).

The multiple unit saddle

Dental implants can be used to stabilise both single crowns and multiple unit fixed prostheses. This section is primarily concerned with situations common to both. The special aspects of single tooth replacement are then discussed.

The technique of treating a patient with an implant-stabilised prosthesis in a bounded or free-end space is essentially the same as for an edentulous patient. A trial appliance is made, a surgeon's guide prepared, implants inserted and a superstructure later fabricated and fitted. The partially edentulous situation nevertheless creates a number of additional problems which must be taken into consideration.

Trial appliance

An important aid when considering possible treatment with an implant-stabilised appliance, or subsequently designing the prosthesis, is a trial appliance. This is similar to that normally used when designing a removable partial denture or fixed bridge, and is usually constructed on an acrylic base. It should be trimmed buccally to represent the final contour of the prosthesis. Where bone resorption has occurred, small flanges can be used to improve the appearance, provided that access for hygiene is adequate. The teeth should be set up to provide a conformative occlusal scheme with full intercuspidation in the intercuspal position. Care must be taken to ensure that there are no interferences in lateral excursions of the jaw. An overcast is then made in silicone elastomer to

aid in visualising the space available, bearing in mind the need for room to clean the appliance.

Surgeon's guide

Armed with this information, the clinician is then in a position to decide on the feasibility of implant treatment. If it is decided to proceed, then a surgeon's guide or template may be prepared. The design of this will depend on access and flap design. It is essential that it can be used during surgery to indicate the positions and orientation of the fixtures. The level of detail of the information which it provides is related to the complexity of the case and the precision required. In partially edentulous patients, the margin of error in implant location is small and the template should therefore be prescriptive. Where a single tooth is replaced, then the guide is usually required to define the position of the fixture. In this application it is preferable if it incorporates a guide for the drill shaft. This ensures that the pilot hole is in precisely the correct site.

Abutment selection

At this stage it is necessary to consider the type of TMA which might be employed. Where the buccal aspect of the saddle will not be visible in normal function then the margins of the bridge abutments can be kept supragingival. This allows the use of a parallel-sided abutment and a small degree of freedom in the antero-posterior positioning of the fixture (**7.9**). In other situations it may be necessary to disguise the abutment by placing the margin of the crown below the mucosal cuff. This requires the use of an abutment with a shoulder and in most systems these are tapered slightly to facilitate crown placement (**7.31–7.33, 7.55–7.57**). This also provides a small amount of freedom in the angulation of the long axis of the crown relative to that of the fixture. Such abutments must be used with a single crown. As a result of the use of this design, the position of the crown is determined precisely by that of the fixture, which must therefore be placed with great care. It must be borne in mind that the majority of fixture designs require a minimum of 6 mm width of ridge into which the fixture is to be inserted, and should be separated from adjacent teeth by at least 2 mm to avoid damaging the periodontal ligament.

Careful thought should be given to the siting of the implant fixture as most designs require a minimum 6 mm width of bone between adjacent teeth, and a separation of at least 3 mm between fixtures.

Bone resorption can result in a change in the contour of the ridge so that if an implant is placed within the bone its long axis would project through the labial face of any crown placed on a straight abutment attached to the fixture. To overcome this problem, some systems employ a range of angulated abutments to provide for the crown being aligned correctly in the arch whilst placing the fixture within the bone. Such abutments may increase the leverage on the joint with the fixture, especially if used with single crowns, and should be used with caution.

Buccal resorption of the alveolus will increase the need to place the implant fixture in a more palatal position. This can make it difficult to place the crown in alignment with the adjacent and opposing natural teeth without creating a ridge lap where cleansing is difficult (7.59), particularly if the crown is to simulate a natural tooth where it emerges through the mucosa.

The depth at which the fixture is placed is also important. It affects not only the location of the crown margin with the abutment but also the shape of the entry profile of the crown within the mucosal tissues. For these reasons, many operators prefer to use healing abutments if these are supplied by the manufacturer. These are slightly wider than the final abutment and therefore facilitate its ultimate placement. They also allow healing of the gingivae to occur before the critical decision as to abutment length is made. Once healing is completed, which usually takes two to three weeks, the healing abutment can be removed. The thickness of the soft tissues is next measured with a special probe and appropriate parallel-sided or tapered abutments installed. When tapered abutments are used their shoulders should lie below the margins of the mucosal cuff.

Surgical stages

The surgical stages for the partially edentulous case are little different in principle to those for the edentulous situation except for the need for considerable precision (7.3–7.6). Care must also be taken not to involve the roots of the natural teeth.

When treating the partially edentulous patient it is not uncommon to find inadequate bone to cover the whole of the implant, especially bucally. This problem is sometimes managed by the technique of guided tissue regeneration, which involves placing the implant in the desired position and accepting the resultant penetration of the bone. A space is then created over the implant in the site where new bone formation is required, for example penetration through a buccal concavity, by placing a micro-perforated membrane over the fixture in this region. This acts as a 'tent' and holds the mucoperiosteum clear of the site, creating a space which fills with a blood clot. The membrane which is most usually employed is a proprietary PTFE product known as Goretex™. Its function is to prevent fibrous tissue formation in the clot which is eventually replaced with bone. It can also prevent epithelial down-growth around the implant and is used in periodontal surgery for this purpose. Once the implant has become surrounded with bone the membrane is removed. Such techniques are likely to become more widely used as patients request implant treatment in locations where there is inadequate bone.

If necessary, the patient will need to be provided with a temporary partial denture whilst integration is taking place. This should be designed to avoid any pressure on the implant sites.

Restorative treatment

Once the soft tissues have healed, the final abutments may be selected and placed as described above. Where healing abutments have been used, this does not usually require a local anaesthetic as they create a slightly oversize space in the soft tissues. The technique used when placing the abutment is the same as that when treating totally edentulous patients.

A temporary bridge prosthesis may then be made, and some manufacturers supply a range of components to help with this. Whilst a prosthesis may be fabricated at the chair side, the procedure is time-consuming and it is preferable to use one made beforehand in the laboratory. This is carried out on a cast prepared from an impression made at the second-stage surgery. Such a bridge will then require only minor modification by the dentist once the abutments have been fitted. Alternatively, the temporary partial denture may be used after suitable modification.

Impression procedures

The impression procedures for the partially edentulous patient are similar to those already described. Lack of room often proscribes the use of screwed impression copings, and a tapered design must be used together with a stiff impression material. A vinyl–siloxane material is suitable. Care must be taken when using this to ensure that all undercuts on the natural teeth which are not required to be recorded are blocked out with carding wax. Failure to observe this precaution can result in the impression locking on the teeth.

The impressions may relate the implants to the dental arch in one of two ways: through either the fixture or the abutment. Frequently, a limited gape prevents the use of copings placed on the abutments, and it is then necessary to use copings placed directly on the fixtures. Whichever technique is used, once the impression has been removed the copings can be dismounted from either the abutments or the fixtures and seated back in the impression. A replica fixture or abutment is then placed on the coping and the cast poured in dental stone to provide an accurate record of the relationship of the fixture to the mucosal cuff and adjacent structures. Some systems allow for the use of parallel-sided screw-retained copings for use on the fixtures and these are withdrawn with the impression after the screws have been removed. It may be advantageous to pour a second cast using a flexible silicone elastomer for the cuff region, as this simplifies abutment selection. The technique is particularly useful where the fixture is deep, as it avoids the problems of fracturing the representation of the cuff on a brittle dental stone cast.

Impressions of the opposing arch are also required, together with the necessary records for mounting the casts on an adjustable articulator.

Verification bar

An acrylic bar should be fabricated in the laboratory so as to be a passive fit on the dummy TMAs (**7.15**). This is then checked in the mouth to confirm the accuracy of the master cast, as described for the treatment of the edentulous case. Some operators like to have the denture teeth set up on this or a similar bar to confirm the appearance of the final appliance. If all is well, then the work is returned to the laboratory for the construction of the cast framework. This is checked in the mouth as for an edentulous case (**7.16–7.18**). The appliance is then ready for completion.

Insertion stage

The appliance should be checked on the articulator and then in the mouth with the fixing screws lightly tightened (**7.23**). The occlusion should be inspected using thin articulating paper to verify that the desired occlusal arrangement has been achieved. There should be even contacts in the intercuspal position of the mandible on both the natural teeth and the prosthesis, and harmony with the adjacent natural teeth in lateral excursions (**7.24–7.26**). Where there are occlusal errors, the prosthesis should be adjusted with fine carborundum stones. Finally, the appliance should be polished, screwed into position and the holes sealed temporarily with light-bodied elastomeric impression material.

Patients must then receive advice on cleaning the prosthesis, which, due to its location, can often be difficult. They should not leave the surgery until they have demonstrated their ability to use appropriate hygiene aids.

Appliance design

The design of the appliance will be dictated by the need to place the artificial teeth in the optimum positions, the requirement for effective hygiene and the strength of the casting (**7.42**). This should follow similar principles to those for an edentulous case.

Occlusal surface material is of importance when opposing natural teeth. Ideally, a material which wears at a similar rate is required; many workers prefer porcelain for this purpose. It has the attractions of being able to provide a pleasing and lasting appearance, and porcelain teeth and gum work can be fired onto a suitable bonding gold alloy in short spans. Gold alloy occlusal surfaces can also provide good service but are often unacceptable due to their unnatural appearance. Polymeric teeth designed for implant use are now made by some manufacturers. They have a large amount of inorganic filler and are claimed to have good wear resistance. If processed onto the metal base with acrylic resin, they have the merit of ease of servicing when worn down.

Whatever type of occlusal surface is selected, the occlusion must be checked regularly as differential wear patterns can give rise to considerable problems if unheeded. These may include over-eruption of opposing teeth and excessive wear and tipping of natural teeth.

Once the clinician and patient are satisfied with the result and a satisfactory level of oral hygiene has been achieved and maintained, the screw holes may be sealed with a thin layer of elastomeric impression material topped with a composite filling material.

Tooth- and implant-stabilised prostheses

The procedure for treatment with these is similar to that outlined above, except that tooth preparation will be required. This follows accepted principles, and could include the use of an adhesive-bonded component, although experience with this configuration is very limited to date. Temporary cementation can be used before the final placing of the bridge; however, once this has been done the potential for subsequent removal for checking is lost.

Linking teeth and implants

The different intrusion stiffness of osseointegrated implants and natural teeth has given rise to concern that the linking of the two with a rigid prosthesis will have unfortunate sequelae. Some workers have suggested that the tooth will become ankylosed due to limited movement. Others have proposed that the bridge will essentially function as a long cantilever and will be prone to fracture.

There is some evidence that the natural tooth may be intruded with resultant cementation failure of the restoration. A possible remedy would be to incorporate a precision attachment in the restoration to allow for some vertical movement at one end or the other; current views tend to favour placing it at the implant end. Laboratory research has provided some support for these points of view and there is limited evidence that teeth with long roots and no abnormal mobility can provide significant support for short fixed bridges linked to implants. Yet clinical opinion at present remains divided and, until sound long-term clinical results are available, there are advantages in avoiding the use of fixed prostheses linking teeth and implants. In any case, the teeth which are used should have long roots, no increased mobility and their periodontal tissues should be healthy.

Hybrid prostheses

Clinical situations sometimes occur where a partially edentulous patient is best treated with an implant-stabilised removable appliance. These can be very stable and provide labial support without the need for surgery to recontour the ridge. They can be designed to cover little gingivae and facilitate oral hygiene in the region of the fixtures as access is good (**7.102–7.105**).

Single tooth prostheses

A single tooth implant is most commonly used to replace a previously extracted incisor tooth and is an alternative choice to a conventional bridge, partial denture or resin-bonded bridge.

The prosthesis typically comprises an implant fixture, a specially designed anti-rotational abutment with an abutment screw and a crown constructed with an aluminous core or a metal alloy base suitable for bonding to porcelain. Excessive loading of the screw joint may cause looseness of the abutment and it is this feature which may limit the use of the prosthesis in other sites within the dental arch. For example, it is unwise to use a single tooth prosthesis which provides canine guidance to the occlusion, whereas group function may be acceptable. Likewise, excessive cantilevering of the crown away from the long axis of the fixture makes it unsuitable for use in premolar or molar sites.

Careful thought should be given to the siting of the implant fixture as most designs require a minimum 6 mm width of bone between adjacent teeth to avoid damage to their periodontal membranes. A similar amount is required labio-lingually if the fixture is to be fully encompassed by bone. The direction of the fixture may therefore be limited both by resorption narrowing the ridge and by the natural alveolar concavity superiorly in the sulcus (**7.75–7.78**).

Inspection of the adjacent natural incisors may also indicate that the natural tooth crowns are not in vertical alignment with, but at an angle to, the long axis of the roots. Preparation of the bony canal for the implant will therefore be required to be in a more vertical plane so that the fixture lies below the cingulum of the crown of the prosthesis (**7.58–7.61**). A straight abutment can then be attached to the fixture with access through the cingulum for passage of the abutment screw. If, in these circumstances, the fixture is placed in a position corresponding with the original root, then the access for the abutment screw will pass through the labial face of the planned crown. An alternative approach used by some systems is to supply an angulated abutment in order to align the crown correctly in the arch whilst placing the fixture within the bone, as described in Chapter 3 (**3.29d**).

Straight abutments are usually formed with a collar and a shoulder, and resistance to rotation is secured against the superior aspect of the fixture by a matched milled surface. In some systems, the internal inferior abutment surface engages the protruding hexagonal top of the fixture and, in others, a protruding octagonal abutment surface passes into the mouth of the fixture. All systems are designed with the intention of providing a smooth junction between abutment and fixture so as to minimise irritation of the soft tissues. Choice of different lengths of collar allows the shoulder on which the crown is formed to be placed 1–2 mm below the margin of the mucosal cuff without the display of metal. The machined hollow cylinder of the abutment above the shoulder and collar (substituting for the core of a crown preparation) provides access for the abutment screw which engages the internal aspect of the fixture uniting abutment to fixture. The abutment cylinder has a minimum length for retention (5 mm) and any excess may be trimmed away to allow the crown to have an appropriate form. This enables a divergence between the long axes of the artificial crown and the fixture to be accommodated, provided that the divergence is not too great (see Chapter 3).

An alternative approach, adopted by some manufacturers, is to use an angulated abutment as this provides an opportunity to correct the divergent alignments of the crown and the fixture. The Calcitek Omnilock system, for example, offers angulations of 15° and 25°. Here the abutment screw passes through the side of the projecting cylinder above the collar. One of several positions for the abutment is possible, so altering the actual alignment to the implant fixture. In this way the position and contour of the crown and its occlusal relationships are most appropriately achieved. This particular Omnilock component may be cut to provide the correct length of cylinder but does not have a shoulder (see Chapter 3).

The Brånemark system employs shouldered abutments and, to ensure maximum stability of the joint between the abutment and fixture, employs a gold alloy screw. Such screws are a potential source of failure in single tooth restorations, and optimum contact is said to exist between this manufacturer's CeraOne abutment and the implant fixture by applying 32 N/cm torque to the screw.

A precisely fitting crown may be achieved with components matched to the abutment. A ceramic core or a plastic burn-out pattern for fabricating a cast alloy backing is available for many systems, allowing a traditional reinforced porcelain crown to be manufactured. Extremes in malpositioning of the fixture, created partly by the volume of available bone, may make difficult the creation of a satisfactory hygienic and aesthetic crown. Palatal positioning of the fixture in a patient with a deep overbite may produce conflict between the abutment and opposing teeth, and as a result steep eccentric incisal guidance upon the crown. Excessive labial positioning of a fixture, corrected with an angulated abutment may, because of the absence of a shoulder, produce a bulky overhang due to the need to produce a minimum 1.5–2 mm thickness of porcelain upon the metal substructure.

Treatment procedures
Surgical procedures

The surgical procedure for insertion of a single tooth implant is no different from that needed for several fixtures.

Various patterns of flap share the common principle of creating a broad base, and an incision involving the adjacent teeth with the capacity to cover the site of penetration and maintain the interdental papillae. With the flap retracted, the relation of the ridge to the template is apparent. Ideally, penetration of bone will often need to follow a more vertical path than the adjacent tooth roots in order to align the fixture beneath the future position of the cingulum of the crown. However, bone resorption after extraction is invariably at the expense of the labial plate and, where less than ideal volume exists, the fixture is positioned more palatally. Where there is a labial concavity, dehiscence during the placement of the fixture is possible and the surgeon may at that stage choose to apply a tissue-regenerating membrane. In the case of the replacement of a central upper incisor, the positioning will be further influenced by the size and location of the incisive fossa. The path of preparation of the bony canal must be very carefully checked to avoid the adjacent periodontal membrane (**7.62–7.71**).

Due to the closeness and height of the adjacent teeth, instruments with long shanks (or the use of an extension tool) are needed to avoid contact with the handpiece when preparing the canal. A long mount may also be needed to place the fixture. Where greater tissue deficiency exists, an earlier surgical procedure of augmentation may be necessary (**7.72–7.74**).

Prosthodontic procedures

Following the second surgical operation at which the healing abutment is attached to the fixture, the partial denture may be adjusted to fit over the abutment and the healing mucosa. When a punch has been used to create a channel, rather than elevation of a flap for access to the cover screw, healing is more rapidly attained and the procedure of adjusting and placing the denture may be adopted immediately or within a few days. The cuff is usually stable, showing no sign of oedema or bleeding after one month.

A primary impression is now recorded in a box tray, using alginate into which a cast is poured. Similarly, an impression is made of the opposing dental arch and this is poured in a die-stone to produce an abrasion-resistant surface to the cast. A shade is also recorded indicating all the variations of hue and characterisation present in the adjacent natural teeth and the crown of the corresponding tooth in the matching quadrant.

Inspection of the primary cast will indicate potential problems which should be discussed with the patient. Difficulties in artificial crown length and width may be anticipated.

It is usually desirable to prepare a special tray constructed over a 2–3 mm spacer of wax into which small channels are cut over teeth in the arch in order to allow stops to be formed on the fitting surface. These ensure the proper positioning of the tray when the impression is made. It is also usual to form a window over the implant site in order to gain access to the impression transfer coping. It is important to avoid unnecessary depth in the design of the flange as this may allow encroachment of a stiff impression material into an alveolar concavity, making difficult the withdrawal of the material from the undercut.

Using a topical anaesthetic to anaesthetise the mucosal cuff, the healing abutment may be unscrewed and the depth of crevice measured from the margin to the fixture head. Usually no soft tissue encroaches across the fixture top. A permanent abutment may next be selected and located upon the fixture head. With the collar of the abutment 1–2 mm below the mucosal cuff, assessment of the relationship with the opposing tooth in the intercuspal position should then reveal a clearance of 2 mm or more. The absence of eccentric interferences with the abutment should also be confirmed (**7.79–7.87**).

Finally, it will be important to examine whether or not the abutment will lie within the intended crown contour as judged in comparison with the adjacent teeth. In order to create a working cast when the abutment is already secured in the mouth with an abutment screw, a matching plastic impression coping is seated upon the implant abutment. Surplus length is cut from its retaining stem and the impression tray is tried in position. An impression recorded in polyether impression material captures the position of the coping. After withdrawal, a plastic replica abutment is fitted into the impression coping and a stone cast is poured. A shallow position of the implant in relation to the cuff will allow this to be poured in improved stone. Where the implant is deeply placed, it is desirable to locate the dummy fixture and pour the cast in two parts. The cuff encircling the tissue adjacent to the teeth and ridge crest is poured in an elastic material (e.g. a silicone elastomer) and the remainder of the master cast is poured in die-stone. This creates a flexible orifice into which the subsequent components of the crown can be fitted without damage to the detail of the cast in the region of the mucosal cuff. Both casts of the jaws are articulated (**7.88–7.91**).

Alternatively, it may be decided to apply a transfer impression coping directly to the fixture head. This procedure will allow the subsequent choice of abutment to be made by the prosthodontist and technician in the laboratory. This is much easier to achieve where the direction or depth of the fixture may require the abutment to be shortened in length, or an angulated style to be used in order to avoid conflict between the face of the crown and the abutment.

When recording the relation of the fixture head to the dental arch, it is more satisfactory to withdraw the transfer coping incorporated in the impression. Use of a technique that requires a tapered coping to be reseated into the impression after its withdrawal from the mouth may allow misalignment within the material. Hence the first step is to place the coping correctly on the fixture hexagon (or into the mouth of the fixture if, for example, the Calcitek Integral System is used). A suitable locating instrument will ensure that the fixture is exactly engaged whilst the fixing screw is tightened. However, if the channel is deep it is wise to record a long cone radiograph to confirm the true positioning of the coping. The special tray is seated with a wax lid to cover the open top, allowing the long screw to perforate the surface. After the application of a suitable fixative, impression material (e.g. polyether elastomer) is loaded and the tray replaced in the mouth. Once

set, the screw is undone and the impression is removed in the direction of the implant fixture. The result should be checked to test the security of the coping and to inspect it to see that no material has passed between the coping and the implant which would indicate its malalignment.

Using the CeraOne component of the Brånemark system, an abutment with appropriate collar length is chosen.

Making the crown

There is now a choice. The crown may be formed upon an aluminous core or with a metal alloy backing, when using CeraOne components. Assuming the abutment is ideally positioned, a suitable core may be chosen and fitted to the dummy abutment or the actual abutment, depending on the technique. Using familiar laboratory procedures, a porcelain crown is built upon the core; first in a biscuit unglazed state and later completed in the glazed state. It is usually wiser to try-in the unglazed crown so that final shaping and the application of stains can be made. After provisional approval has been given by the patient, the final glazing of the crown is carried out (**7.92**).

When a porcelain fused to metal technique is selected, a preformed plastic pattern is fitted to the abutment in the laboratory. Inlay casting wax is added and an entire crown formed. Next, the crown is indexed on the labial surface in silicone putty to record the ideal labial contour. The wax is then cut back so that the correct bulk will be given to the areas in which porcelain is to be added. It is essential to examine both intercuspal and eccentric relations of the backing and the crown to avoid premature occlusal contact. Such contacts are likely to overstress the abutment screw joint (**7.93**).

The backing is invested and cast in a suitable gold-content gold/palladium alloy. After cleaning and polishing, an opaque layer is fired onto the backing before building up the remainder of the neck, body and incisal edge of the crown. When shaping the crown, it is preferable to be able to create the ideal emergence angle without ridge lap or excess labial bulk.

Before examining the trial crown, it is essential to be certain that the selected abutment is accurately positioned and fully seated. Confirmation using a long cone X-ray is essential. The abutment screw may then be tightened optimally. When using a gold alloy CeraOne screw 32 N/cm is the recommended torque to be applied by the mechanical driver, using a torque controller to avoid excessive forces on the implant and bone interface.

Fitting the crown

After glazing the porcelain, the metal backing will require re-polishing before the crown is cemented. It should be appreciated that components are a precise fit so that excess amounts of cement or the use of a mix of viscous consistency or advanced set will prevent the crown from being correctly seated. The length and occlusion of the crown will then be incorrect. Added to this problem is the important matter of displacing the cuff with sufficient force to allow the crown to be seated. It is wise, therefore, to apply correctly mixed temporary cement during placement of the crown with a positive seating pressure. The crown may be radiographed again to check the exactness of fit once surplus set material is removed from the crevice. Most operators would consider that a proprietary zinc-oxide-based temporary cement is sufficient to produce an effective lute. A crown may more easily be seated if there is a manufactured space above the abutment for the surplus of luting medium. Also, it may be more easily withdrawn if a ledge is fashioned in the cingulum on which an instrument may be used to exert a withdrawal force. Pressure against the crown margin is, of course, likely to damage the porcelain border. It is essential to check the occlusion to ensure that premature occlusal contacts are avoided. Adjustments should be made using Shimstock, ultra-thin articulating paper or occlusal indicator wax placed between both arches to identify such contacts. This corrective procedure will help to avoid the generation of excessive occlusal loads upon the crown (**7.94–7.97**).

It is important to advise the patient to avoid excessive forces between the prosthesis and the opposing teeth. Also, the capacity of the patient to clean the cuff and the interproximal spaces using a brush and Superfloss must be assessed after an appropriate period of instruction.

The particular problem of seating the crown may be significantly reduced in one of two ways. It is possible to replace a traditional 4 mm diameter healing abutment with a larger custom-made component devised to expand the cuff to an appropriate entry to receive the ideal bullet-shaped crown. Alternatively, a temporary crown may be constructed in acrylic resin using a temporary post upon the abutment. It is then easier to maintain the orifice of the cuff in the correct form, as well as providing an opportunity for producing the best shape once the mucosa has reached a fully healed state.

Not all of the problems of restoring a pleasing appearance are overcome easily. It is wise to attempt to identify them before treatment with a diagnostic wax-up (**7.98–7.101**).

SUMMARY OF TREATMENT PHASES FOR SINGLE TOOTH FIXED IMPLANT PROSTHESES: INCISOR CROWN

Phase 1: Record primary impressions
- Record primary impressions over healing abutment and of the opposing arch.

Phase 2: Design special tray
- Provide access for impression transfer coping and passage for fixing screw.

Method A
Phase 3: Position abutment
- Remove healing abutment and measure mucosal cuff depth to fixture.
- Select abutment with a collar that lies 1–2 mm below the orifice.
- Check the occlusion provides ≥2 mm clearance.
- Confirm the abutment top lies within the expected body of the planned crown.
- Secure the abutment with the abutment screw (32 N/cm for gold alloy screw of the Brånemark CeraOne system).
- Record long cone intra-oral radiograph, confirming fit.

Phase 4: Position abutment impression transfer coping
- Place plastic transfer coping onto the CeraOne abutment.
- Shorten the stem.
- Insert impression tray, check fit and extension with clearance for coping.
- Seal wax lid, apply adhesive, record polyether impression.
- Withdraw impression and fit replica plastic abutment to coping.

Phase 5: Pour master cast
- Apply 0.1 mm wax film to a depth of 2 mm along the replica from the impression surface to create a thin relief.
- Pour the cast in improved dental stone.
- Withdraw the impression.
- Fit another coping to the replica abutment in the cast and make an index using laboratory putty silicone elastomer.
- Withdraw the index and perforate it in two sites with a 2 mm diameter rose-head bur.
- Cut back the cast to expose the replica abutment collar or fixture head.

- Reseat the silicone index (after the application of an ultra-thin coat of petroleum jelly).
- Pour in Gingifast silicone to rebuild the cuff surrounding the fixture.

Phase 6: (see below).

Method B
Phase 3: Position fixture transfer coping
- Remove healing abutment and localise an impression transfer coping (single tooth type) directly onto the fixture, securing it in place with the fixing screw.
- Insert the impression tray, check extension, fit and clearance for the coping.
- Seal with a wax lid, apply adhesive and record a polyether impression.
- Withdraw impression and attach replica fixture to the coping.

Phase 4: Pour master cast
- Use same principles as for phase 5, method A.
- Add wax film along the fixture replica for 2 mm.
- Pour cast and remove impression.
- Fit another transfer coping and make a silicone index.
- Release fixing screw, remove and cut back cast.
- Pour a silicone cuff surrounding fixture.

Phase 5: Position abutment
- Select an abutment with a collar which lies 1–2 mm below the orifice of the silicone cuff; confirm the occlusal space and length are suitable (see phase 3, method A).

Phase 6: Construct a metal-bonded crown
- Fit a preformed plastic pattern to the abutment.
- Wax-up a crown to the required shape.
- Make a labial index.
- Check the occlusion, avoiding premature contact.
- Cut back the pattern to form a backing, leaving the correct space for porcelain.
- Cast the backing in gold/palladium alloy.
- Build the porcelain crown.

Phase 6 (alternative): Construct an aluminous-cored porcelain crown

- Select an aluminous core, fit to the abutment and correct the occlusion, if needed.
- Build a porcelain crown and fire to unglazed state.

Phase 7: Trial insertion

- Position crown, displacing the mucosal cuff.
- Confirm shade, shape and fit.
- Confirm contact points, absence of premature occlusal contacts.

Phase 8: Fit crown

- Stain and glaze crown.
- Confirm fit of the abutment.
- Check security of abutment screw if the design employs one. Record long cone radiograph to check fit.
- Seal access hole with temporary material (e.g. gutta percha).
- Cement with a temporary cement.

Phase 9: Reassess crown

- Examine security of fit and occlusion of the crown.
- Monitor the oral hygiene standard.

SUMMARY OF TREATMENT PHASES FOR MULTI-UNIT FIXED BRIDGE IMPLANT PROSTHESES

Many of the procedures for this treatment are almost identical to those described in Chapters 5 and 6. The section above describes the use of abutments designed for single crowns, which may be used for some or all of the abutments, depending on the appearance to be produced by the final prosthesis.

Phase 1: Record primary impressions
- Record primary impressions over either healing abutments or tapered impression copings.
- Record impression of the opposing arch.

Phase 2: Design special tray
- Decide on coping type. In anterior saddles it is often possible to gain access to screw-retained copings. More posteriorly the gape may not permit this and tapered coping must then be used. Provide access for impression transfer coping and passage for fixing screw when necessary.

Phase 3: Position abutments
- Remove healing abutment and measure mucosal cuff depth to fixture.
- If using tapered abutments, select one with a collar that lies 1–2 mm below the orifice of the mucosal cuff.
- If using parallel-sided abutments choose one which will project 2 mm above mucosal cuff. Longer abutments may be needed; refer to diagnostic appliance or try-in.
- Check that the occlusion provides ≥2 mm clearance.
- Confirm that the abutment top lies within the expected body of the planned bridge.
- Secure the abutment using the appropriate technique (design-dependent).
- Record long cone intra-oral radiograph, confirming fit.

Phase 4: Record impressions
- Record working impression of abutments, and impression of opposing arch.

- Where possible, record jaw relationship for mounting casts. If numbers of teeth are inadequate for this, construct record block and base for next visit.
- Record shade of teeth.

Phase 5: Construct check bar
- Construct check bar and trial appliance.

Phase 6: Try-in
- Confirm master cast using trial bar.
- Use trial partial denture to confirm positions, appearance and arrangement of teeth.

Phase 7: Verify casting

- Confirm shape and fit of cast framework.

Phase 8: Construction of prosthesis
- Complete construction of prosthesis.

Phase 9: Insertion of prosthesis
- Insert prosthesis and check carefully the fit of the gold cylinders.
- Check and adjust occlusion as necessary.
- Confirm that patient knows how to keep prosthesis clean.

Phase 10: Review
- Recheck occlusion. At intervals of 1 to 1.5 years, the bridge should be removed and the status of the implants and surrounding tissues checked.
- Monitor oral hygiene.

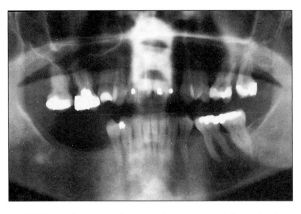

7.1 This patient requires replacement of the missing mandibular teeth on the right.

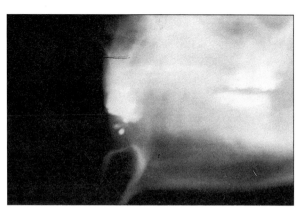

7.2 A trial denture incorporating ball bearings as markers was used with a series of tomograms to confirm the feasibility of inserting implants.

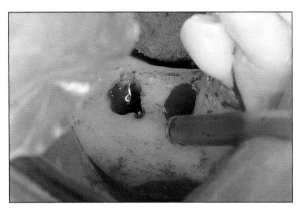

7.3 Using a surgical template, the mandible was exposed and the fixture sites prepared.

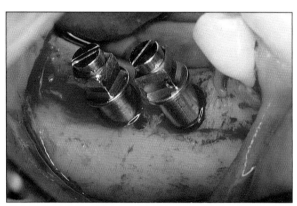

7.4 Brånemark fixtures have been placed and are shown here with their mounts.

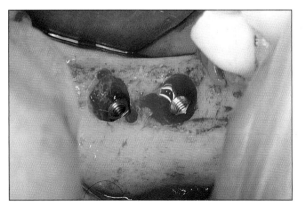

7.5 The mounts have been removed and the fixtures can be observed in the bone.

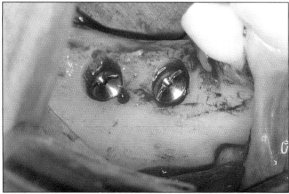

7.6 Cover screws have been placed on the fixtures.

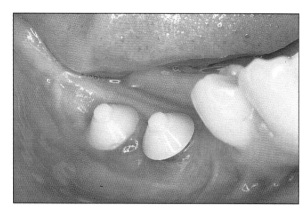

7.7 The appearance of the implant site two weeks after second-stage surgery. Large healing caps are in place.

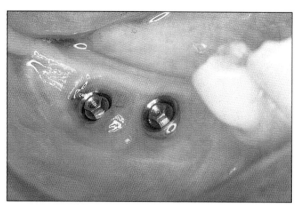

7.8 After removal of the healing caps it is evident that the distal abutment is too short.

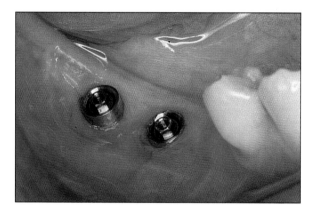

7.9 A longer abutment has been placed on the distal fixture.

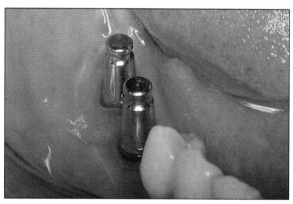

7.10 Tapered impression copings have been screwed on to the implant abutment; a primary impression is then recorded in alginate in a stock impression tray.

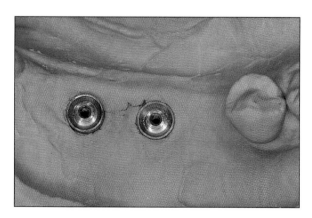

7.11 The primary cast incorporating replica abutments.

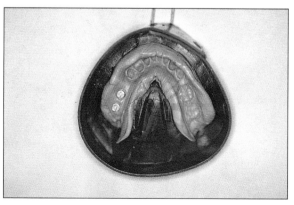

7.12 A working impression is recorded in elastomer and then boxed ready for pouring. The replica abutments mounted on the tapered impression copings can be seen.

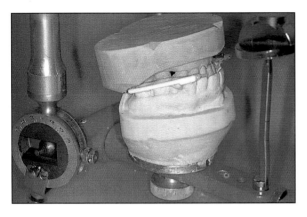

7.13 The master cast is mounted on an adjustable articulator using an inter-occlusal record.

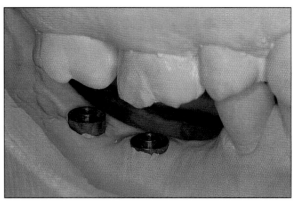

7.14 The relationship of the opposing natural teeth to the replica abutments can be seen on these casts.

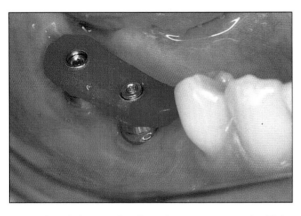

7.15 A trial acrylic bar is constructed. This incorporates gold cylinders, and is checked in the mouth to confirm the accuracy of the master cast.

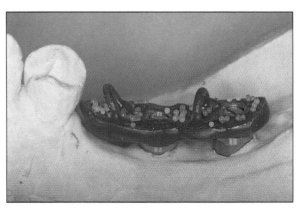

7.16 A metal framework for the prosthesis is then waxed up.

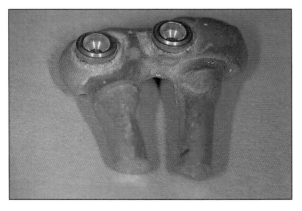

7.17 The framework as cast showing the gold cylinders which have become incorporated into the gold alloy.

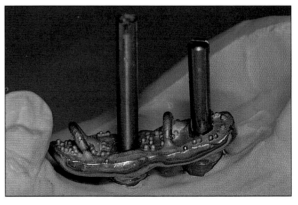

7.18 The finished framework is checked on the master cast.

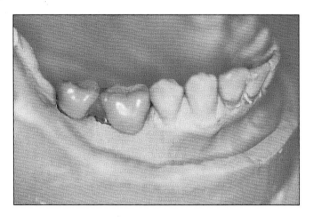

7.19 Teeth are then waxed up on the framework.

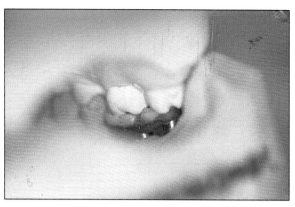

7.20 It is important to check the occlusal relationships of the trial appliance lingually as well as buccally.

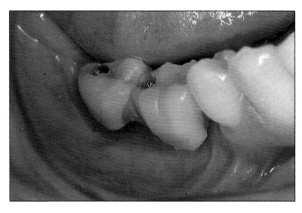

7.21 The trial appliance is checked in the mouth to confirm the positions of the teeth.

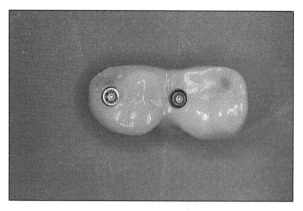

7.22 The finished prosthesis. The gold cylinder screws can be seen in the holes in the occlusal surface.

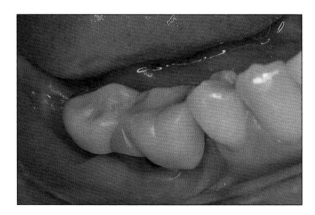

7.23 The appliance is then placed in the mouth and, after checking and adjusting, the occlusion is fixed in position and the screw holes sealed with rubber bungs and a composite resin.

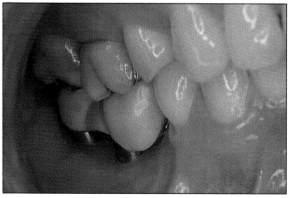

7.24 The occlusal relationships of the bridge in the inter-cuspal position.

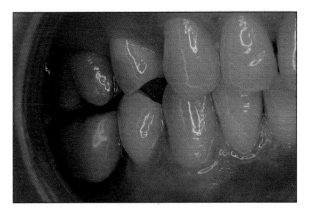

7.25 The fixed bridge prosthesis loses occlusal contacts in right lateral excursions due to canine guidance.

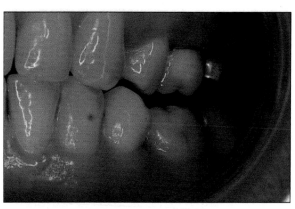

7.26 Occlusal contacts on the prosthesis will also be lost in left lateral excursions due to canine guidance. This avoids non-working side interferences.

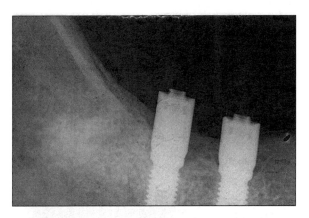

7.27 Radiograph of the completed case at one year.

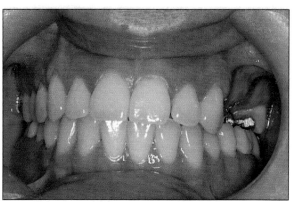

7.28 This patient has a bounded space in the right maxilla which is to be restored with an implant-stabilised fixed prosthesis.

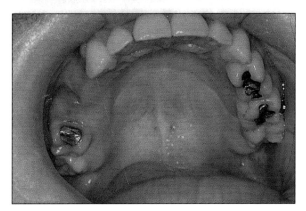

7.29 Occlusal view of the space to be restored.

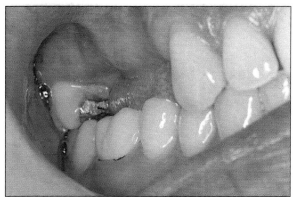

7.30 Buccal view of the space to be restored.

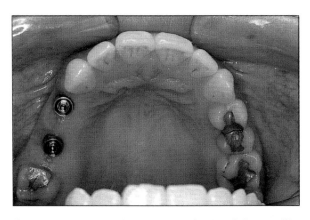

7.31 Implants have been placed in the right maxilla and tapered abutments mounted on them.

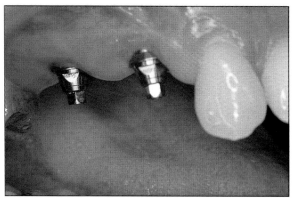

7.32 Buccal view of the tapered abutments showing their relationship to the mucosal cuff.

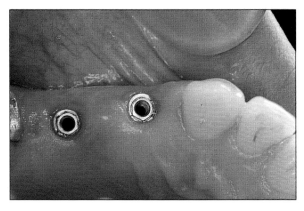

7.33 Occlusal view of the tapered abutments. Bone contours prevented their buccal shoulders being placed below the mucosal cuff.

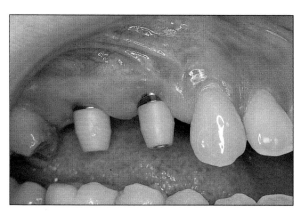

7.34 Healing caps have been placed on the tapered abutments.

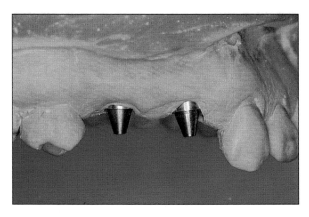

7.35 Master cast showing the abutment replicas.

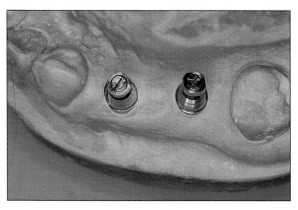

7.36 Conical gold cylinders have been placed on the abutment replicas.

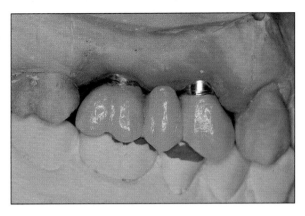

7.37 The completed porcelain-faced bridge.

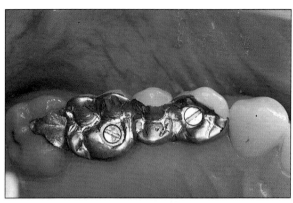

7.38 Occlusal view of the completed prosthesis.

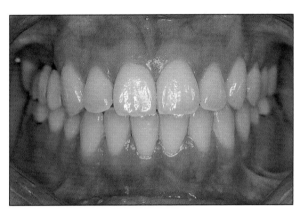

7.39 Anterior view of the completed reconstruction.

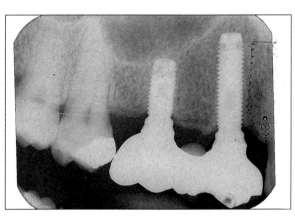

7.40 Radiograph of the implants one year after completion of treatment.

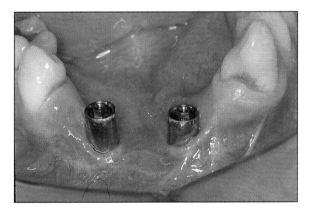

7.41 This patient had lost his anterior mandibular teeth and a considerable amount of supporting bone in a road traffic accident. Two implants were used with parallel-sided abutments to stabilise a fixed prosthesis.

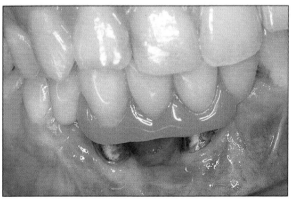

7.42 The prosthesis at the trial stage. Considerable clearance has been left below the appliance to aid oral hygiene. This gap cannot be seen except when the lip is retracted.

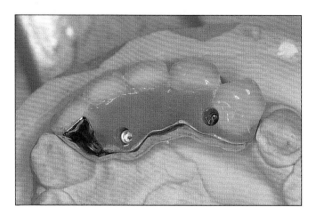

7.43 Occlusal view of the completed appliance on the master cast.

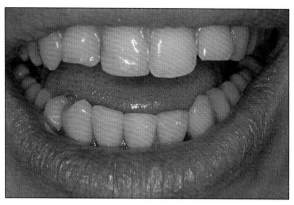

7.44 Anterior view of the completed restoration.

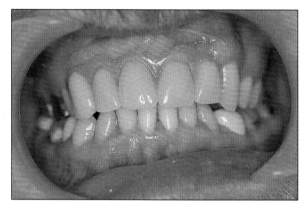

7.45 Partial fixed prosthesis inserted to restore a long anterior span in the maxillary arch.

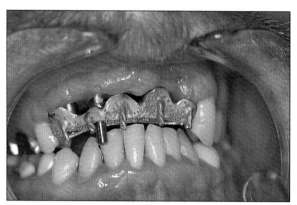

7.46 Cast metal frame tried in position.

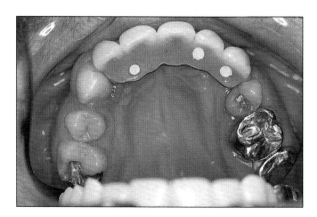

7.47 Palatal view of fixed partial prosthesis fitted to replace a partial denture.

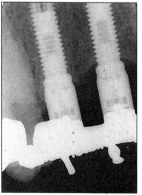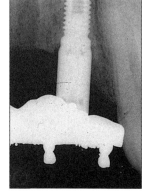

7.48 Two periapical radiographs showing bone levels after four years.

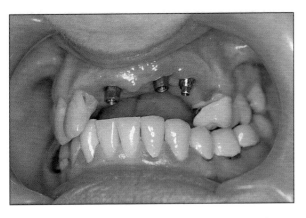

7.49 Two tapered shouldered abutments and one single tooth abutment *in situ*, showing divergence of alignment.

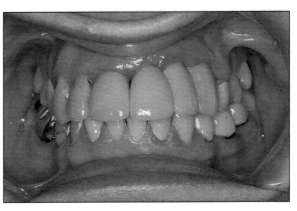

7.50 Newly inserted porcelain–metal fixed partial prosthesis and a single tooth prosthesis. Note the increased crown lengths provided by the reduction of bone associated with the traumatic loss of teeth.

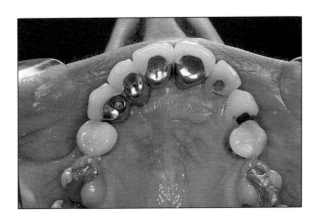

7.51 Palatal view of the restored arch.

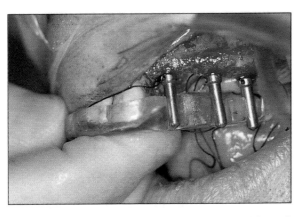

7.52 Surgical template confirming the position of bony canals using direction indicators.

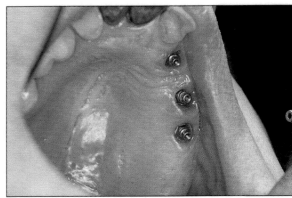

7.53 Tapered shouldered abutments in place.

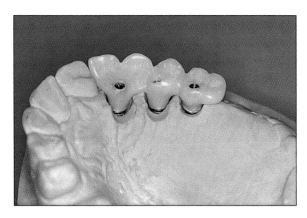

7.54 Temporary prosthesis prepared for case.

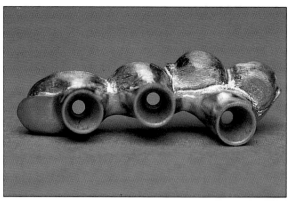

7.55 Cast metal frame enclosing tapered (Nobelpharma Estheticone) cylinders.

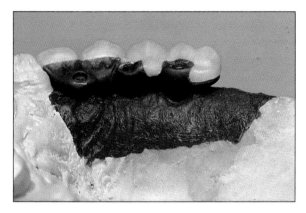

7.56 Completed metal ceramic fixed prosthesis on laboratory cast. Silicone replicates the mucosal cuffs.

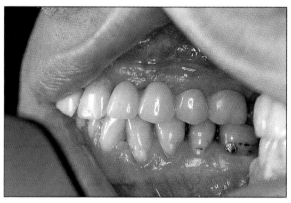

7.57 Distal extension fixed prosthesis in place.

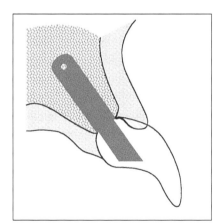

7.58 Diagram illustrating a fixture ideally related to the crown.

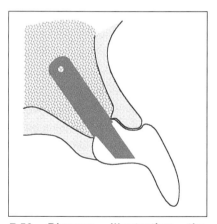

7.59 Diagram illustrating the production of a ridge lap of the crown as a result of the palatal position of the implant fixture within the resorbed ridge.

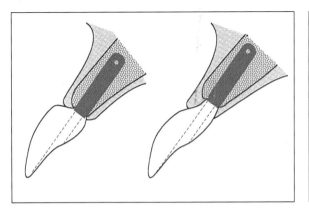

7.60 Diagram illustrating a more superior apical position for the fixture which enhances the entry profile of the crown in the mucosal cuff.

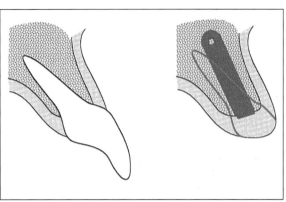

7.61 Diagram illustrating the means of creating a straight implant linkage between the abutment and the fixture. The fixture is planned to be sited more vertically than the extracted tooth root.

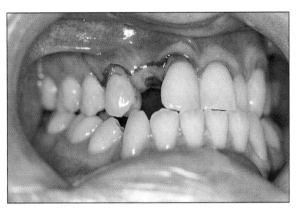

7.62 Line of incision and the position of the implant marked initially.

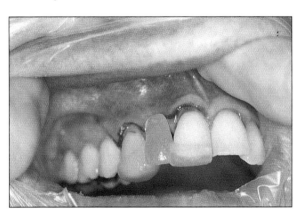

7.63 Template used to guide the surgeon in choosing an implant position within the labial contour of the crown.

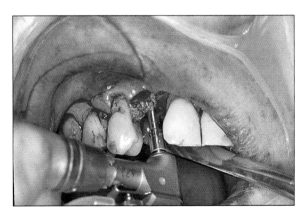

7.64 Utilising the pilot drill within the initial penetration of the alveolus.

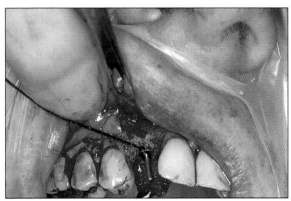

7.65 Checking that the direction of the bony canal is suitable for placement of the crown. Note the retaining suture to avoid accidental loss of the indicator.

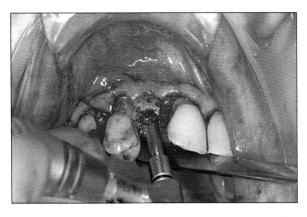

7.66 A spade drill used to gouge bone to the required diameter of the implant fixture.

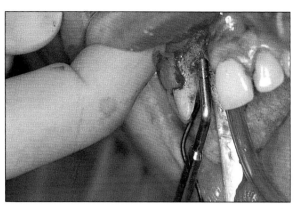

7.67 Graduated gauge may be used to determine the depth of the bony canal to assist the selection of a fixture of appropriate length.

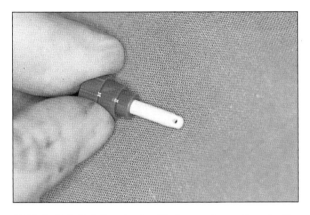

7.68 A Calcitek implant withdrawn from the sterile capsule.

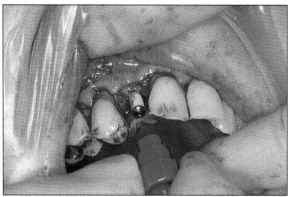

7.69 Inserting the hydroxyapatite-coated implant.

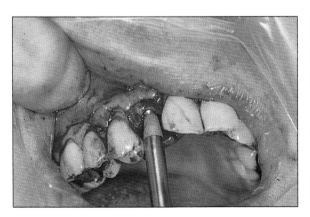

7.70 Seating the implant in the canal.

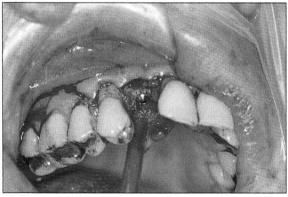

7.71 Cover screw sealing the orifice of the implant before closure of the flap.

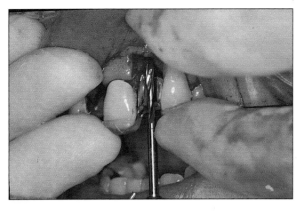

7.72 Either a long shank or an extension for mounting a twist drill is necessary when preparing a canal in a narrow span of the dental arch.

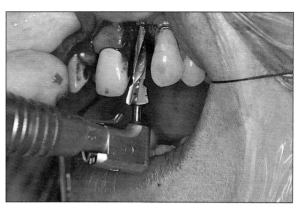

7.73 Sufficient space must exist for the countersink drill. Here an extension is required to avoid a clash with the handpiece.

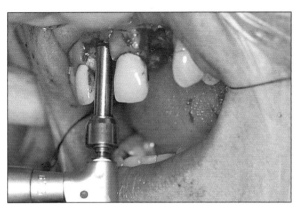

7.74 Using a long fixture mount to ensure adequate clearance for the connector holding the fixture mount.

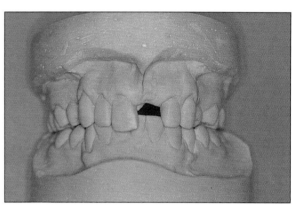

7.75 Study cast showing site of an extracted upper incisor tooth having a favourable incisor overbite.

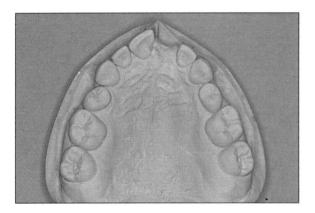

7.76 Study cast illustrating the width available between the adjacent teeth and in the alveolar process.

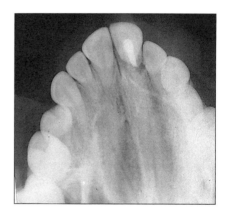

7.77 Anterior occlusal X-ray showing resorption of the left central incisor root.

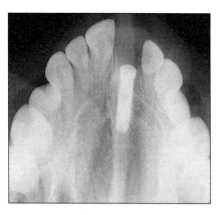

7.78 Anterior occlusal X-ray showing implant fixture engaging the floor of nose and avoiding the incisive canal.

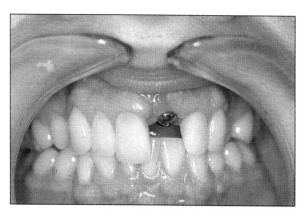

7.79 Healing abutment placed at surgical stage 2, with the mucosal cuff healed after three weeks.

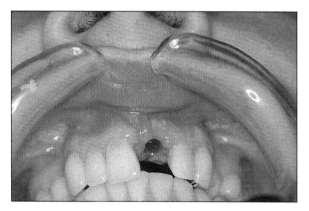

7.80 Channel created in the alveolar mucosa by removing the healing abutment.

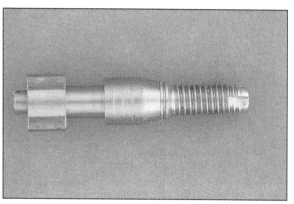

7.81 A transfer impression coping secured to the hexagonal top of an implant fixture.

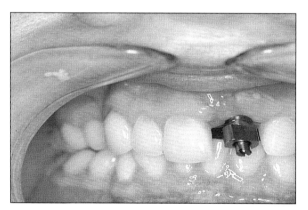

7.82 Transfer impression coping secured upon the fixture with an appropriate fixing screw, *in situ*.

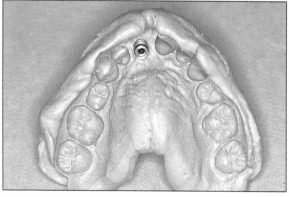

7.83 Completed impression withdrawing the impression coping from the fixture, within the polyether impression.

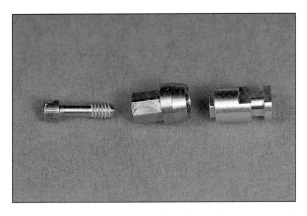

7.84 Dummy fixture with CeraOne abutment and gold alloy abutment screw for use with the Brånemark system.

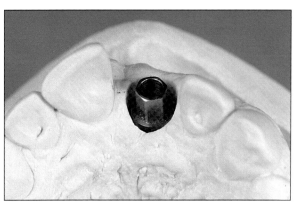

7.85 A master cast incorporating a dummy fixture on which is seated a titanium CeraOne abutment with a collar length suitable to place the shoulder 1 mm below the margin of the mucosal cuff.

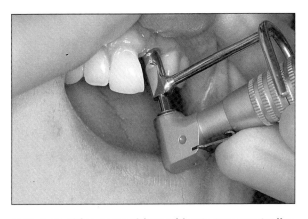

7.86 A machine screwdriver with a torque controller may be used to secure the abutment screw. The driver passes through a miniature tubular spanner which fits over the abutment. The yoke fitting around the handpiece prevents rotation of the abutment when the screw is tightened.

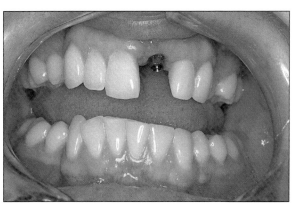

7.87 The shouldered abutment *in situ*.

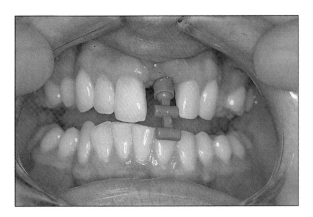

7.88 Plastic impression coping in place upon the abutment.

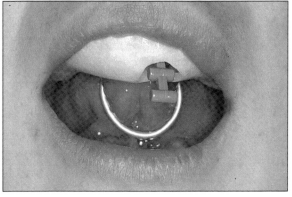

7.89 Special impression tray tried in the mouth to examine the clearance for the coping which may be linked with self-cure resin to the tray when the impression material has set.

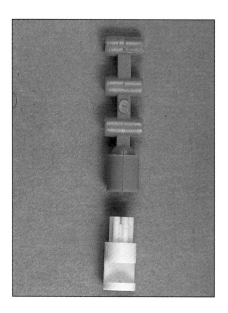

7.90 Replica plastic abutment (yellow) and (blue) plastic transfer coping for use with the Brånemark system.

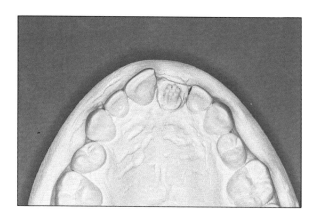

7.91 Master cast poured from a working impression incorporating a plastic abutment, as an alternative to using a titanium abutment.

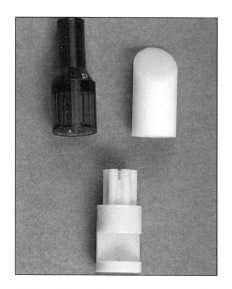

7.92 Alternative choices for providing the core of a porcelain single tooth crown. A blue plastic burn-out pattern forms the basis of a metal-bonded crown. An aluminous cone may substitute for the core of an 'all porcelain' crown.

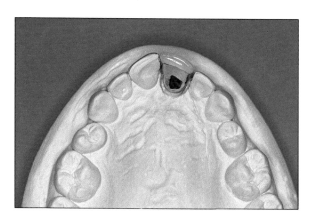

7.93 The cast metal substructure of a porcelain-bonded crown.

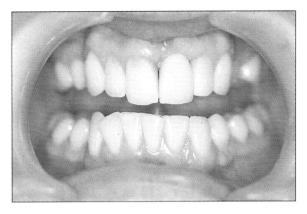

7.94 The single tooth crown tried-in on the abutment after the porcelain has been fired to a 'biscuit bake'.

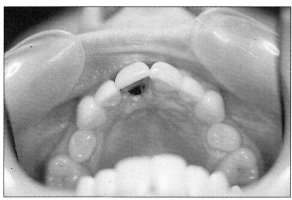

7.95 Occlusal view of the single tooth crown cemented in position.

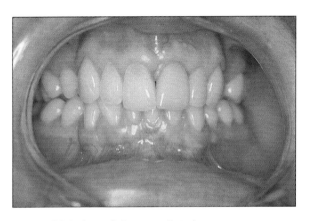

7.96 Labial view of the completed crown.

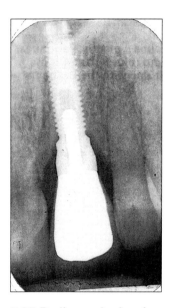

7.97 Radiograph showing the completed crown with the abutment secured to the fixture by a gold alloy screw. Monitored at 18 months after cementation of the crown.

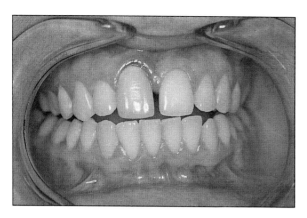

7.98 A failing post crown on a natural tooth.

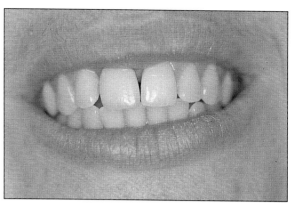

7.99 At the request of the patient the median diastema has been closed with the construction of a single tooth crown. The gingival margin is not evident during a smile.

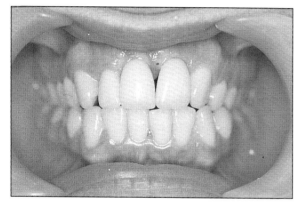

7.100 Two single tooth crowns cemented on Omniloc conical abutments of the Calcitek System. Loss of the gingival papillae is barely noticeable.

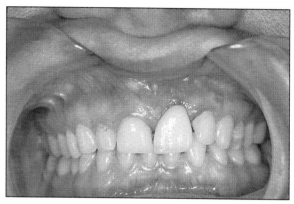

7.101 An unfavourable appearance created by a combination of deficiency of tissue and the positioning of the fixture avoiding the incisive fossa.

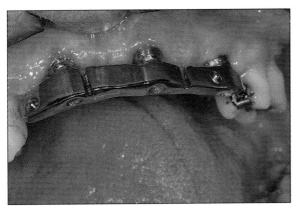

7.102 Where it is inappropriate to employ ridge augmentation techniques, correct tooth positions and labial support can be provided using an implant-stabilised removable appliance. This patient's prosthesis is stablised by a milled bar attached to three fixtures.

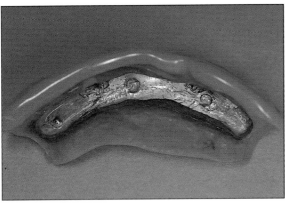

7.103 The fitting surface of the prosthesis showing the cast gold sleeve. This is located by grooves and retained by friction and two precision attachments placed horizontally in the bar. These have spring-loaded plungers which engage dimples in the palatal aspect of the sleeve.

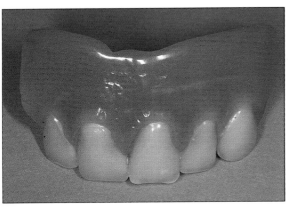

7.104 The labial aspect of the prosthesis.

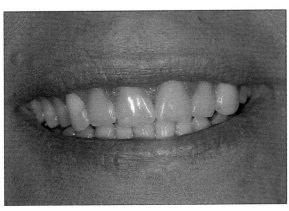

7.105 The prosthesis in place.

8. Maxillo-Facial Prostheses

Introduction

Facial deformity arising from congenital disorders, severe trauma and the excision of tumours of the jaws, skull and face is frequently managed by several experts. In some instances, such as the treatment of congenital cleft lip and palate, restoration requires the combined care of maxillo-facial or plastic surgeons and orthodontists to create a harmonious outcome in the resulting appearance and function of the repaired soft-tissue deformity of the face overlying the corrected bony skeleton and dental arch.

The entire procedure for a localised defect may be in the hands of the plastic surgeon when, for instance, reconstruction of a microtic ear is planned. However, not all situations can be treated partially or totally with surgery, so that suitable rehabilitation may call for the provision of a removable facial prosthesis. This may be 'free standing' or linked to oral prostheses depending upon the site, size of defect and need for mutual stability created by the interlocking of two or more parts.

Traditional methods of fixation of a facial prosthesis rely on less than ideal solutions. The use of elastics and spectacle frames to retain a 'hard' acrylic resin device may produce excessive pressure upon the skin, which is more prone to ulceration after radiotherapy treatment. Failure of movement of the margin of the prosthesis will make the result even less satisfactory when the patient speaks and smiles. However, whilst the use of resilient elastomers producing a flexible lightweight prosthesis may overcome these problems, retention is often achieved with contact adhesives that may cause irritation to the skin. Regular removal will promote tearing of the fine knife-edge margins which blend with the facial contours.

The introduction of implants to restore the dentition has been extended to maxillo-facial rehabilitation and so solve many of the problems created by a deficient biomechanical link.

Traditionally designed dental implant fixtures may therefore be positioned in the root of the zygoma, palatal vault, nasal floor and pterygoid regions either to stabilise a dental obturator prosthesis or to provide anchorage for a facial prosthesis.

A different design of implant is appropriate for use in the skull in the regions of the mastoid bone, supra-orbital and lateral orbital rim, and below the anterior nasal spine in the region of the columella (**8.1**). In order to avoid penetration to vital structures (e.g. the sigmoid sinus in the mastoid region) and gain sufficient anchorage, the fixture (of 3 or 4 mm depth and 3.75 mm diameter) is constructed with a flange which engages a recess surgically prepared in the cortical plate. Each perforation in the flange acts to engage the bony surface and so significantly increases the stability of short length fixture in the bony canal and the subsequent area of osseointegration (**8.2–8.5**).

Additional use can be made of this type of fixture to support a hearing aid for those patients with conductive deafness. This aid has been developed by Nobelpharma to couple into a special abutment, enabling the patient to position or withdraw the aid with an easy movement. Hence the placement of one additional implant will allow rehabilitation of the appearance with an ear prosthesis and the enhancement of hearing with a secure bone-anchored aid (**8.6, 8.7**).

More extensive and difficult replacement may be sought where both facial and oral tissues require rehabilitation with a combination of linked prostheses which apply considerable stress to the interfaces existing between bone and traditional dental and specialised skull implants. Moreover, there may also be a need to prepare the site of facial reconstruction by autogenous bone grafting and by soft-tissue reconstruction with myocutaneous flaps or full thickness and split skin grafting, prior to the placement of implants. Reports of the results of these forms of treatment relate to much shorter periods of observation in limited numbers of patients. Early indications are that different levels of success will be achieved in different sites of the facial skeleton and will be influenced by the use of radiotherapy employed in the treatment of a malignancy. The introduction of hyperbaric oxygen therapy for these cases suggests that considerable improvement in the outcome is possible.

Due to the complexity of treatment there is a need for collaborative effort by a team (surgeon, prosthodontist, maxillo-facial technician) to provide maxillo-facial treatment. They will have, when needed, the assistance of an expert operating theatre nurse, plastic surgeon, audiological physician, clinical psychologist and dental hygienist.

Surgical assessment is necessary to determine the quantity and quality of bone available for the placement of implant fixtures, together with information about the overlying skin and mucosa which the abutments will ultimately penetrate. Estimation of the difficulty of access to each site is needed to ensure that surgical instrumentation and prosthetic attachment are feasible. Evaluation of the available bone is achieved from a CT scan, and depths may be gauged from reformatted images produced, for example, as 2 mm contiguous slices (**8.8a, 8.8b**). In order to achieve a healthy cuff of skin around the abutments, it may be necessary to plan to reduce sub-epithelial tissue in order to create a thin non-mobile cuff which is attached over a 0.5 mm radius around the abutment or to remove hair-bearing skin and graft skin taken from a hairless region.

The prosthodontist has the responsibility of defining the likely border of the prosthesis and ensuring, where feasible, that the margin is applied to non-mobile areas of the face and that it is in harmony with the contours created by folds in the skin or bony anatomy.

A plan for the expected anchorage sites should locate the abutment within the expected border of the prosthesis. There must be sufficient depth to accommodate the retentive components including the acrylic resin substructure.

Assessment of the expected loads and resistance to the consequent directions of displacement is needed to determine whether or not implants require to be linked or may stand alone.

Particular problems of colouration to match the skin and requirements to incorporate hair, eyebrows, lashes etc. to enhance the disguise should be determined by the maxillo-facial technician.

General surgical principles and techniques

Production of an ear prosthesis

Successful replacement of the ear is achieved by the construction of a silicone prosthesis retained by a minimum of two skull implants positioned in the mastoid process. The prosthesis is then clipped to a bar screwed to the implant abutments.

The general principles of case planning apply to this situation and great care must be taken in cases of congenital deformity. This is because facial asymmetry and variations in thickness of the skull make the positioning of implants more difficult than in cases with little local distortion of the soft tissues and normal thickness of the skull (**8.9**).

Clinical appraisal is required to determine the position of the tip of the mastoid process and to relate this structure to the external auditory canal and tragus, if present. Inspection will also determine the site of movement of the skin as the

condyle shifts on opening and closing of the mouth, and hence the likely limit of the anterior margin of the prosthesis. Local scarring and the position of soft-tissue remnants (e.g. lobe) and residual cartilage are considered in relation to the site of the prosthesis (**8.10, 8.11**). An impression is recorded of the normal ear without distortion using a mix of alginate with double the water to powder ratio. An impression is similarly made of the side of the face, on which are previously marked suitable reference lines (e.g. Frankfurt plane), and stone models are poured (**8.12**).

The maxillo-facial technician will next prepare a replica ear in wax, either by modelling upon the stone cast or by recording an impression of another patient's ear of similar shape into which wax may be poured directly (**8.13**). Also, he may construct a clear acrylic resin template to fit the affected site. The wax ear is positioned on the affected side of the face, being compared for level, prominence and antero-posterior position (**8.14–8.16**). When this is judged to be correct, two or three possible implant sites below the anthelix, which is the thickest part of the external ear, may be marked on the skin. These are usually found to be 20 mm from the centre of the external auditory meatus, commonly at 2 and 4 o'clock on the left hand side of the face and at 8 and 10 upon the right side. The position of the ear is recorded by outlining the perimeter or the insertion points of the ear. The clear template is then placed over the face and marked with the proposed positions for the implants. When an implant is to be positioned for a hearing aid, the site should be identified 2 cm distal to the helix within the hairline. Determination of the thickness of the skull may be required using a CT scan, across the mastoid about the middle third of the face (**8.17, 8.18**).

It may be appropriate to mark the skin, before scanning, with an adherent 2 mm diameter radiopaque disc over each site. Direct readings of the skull thickness at 2 cm distance from the auditory canal can be made in order to confirm this likely suitability. The surgeon now has the means of placing implants in the most appropriate site to secure a good cosmetic effect from the prosthesis, provided the template can be accurately located at the commencement of the surgical operation for installing the fixtures.

Surgical technique

Percutaneous implant placement is completed under full aseptic technique and invariably under general anaesthesia. The operation is preceded by clinically evaluating the appropriate siting for implant placement relative to the local anatomy, the altered symmetry of the face in developmental anomalies and the awareness of the ultimate perforation sites relative to hair-bearing skin and facial tissue movement.

Hair is bacteriologically dirty and is shaved preoperatively. Some mark indicating the leading edge of the temporal hairline is helpful. The ideal implant sites, as determined by the template, are marked through the skin and onto the cranial bone pre-operatively. The site is liberally infiltrated with local anaesthesia (1% lignicaine with 1/200 000 adrenaline added) and covered with Steridrape to reduce the transference of skin pathogens.

A curved incision 1–2 cm to one side of the proposed implant sites is made to periosteum and the use of diathermy (bipolar) minimised. Flap mobility is developed. The dye pricked through the skin already injected at optimum proposed sites may be seen staining periosteum and membrane (**8.19**).

Sharp periosteal dissection 1.5 cm to one side of the proposed implant site allows reflection of that layer and identification of the superior temporal line, the mastoid process and the descent into the external auditory meatus at the supramental spine (**8.20**).

The sequential use of cutting tools, starting with a rose-head bur, establishes the texture of the bone and is continued until the shoulder of the bur meets the bone. The longest possible shaft is sunk (preferably 4 mm). To go through mastoid air cells is normal, to meet dura is not unusual but it is advisable to avoid the sigmoid sinus. All are low-pressure systems and perforation of the dura or a venous sinus can be dealt with by a muscle plug.

The channels are tapped with a titanium screw tap, but experience has shown that soft bone does not need to be pre-tapped and the initial entry of the flanged fixture as a self-tap manoeuvre provides a more stable immobilisation (**8.21–8.24**).

The hexagonal format of the implant is covered by a cover screw, or the central screw hole obliterated by a spacer screw if the overlying skin is thin. The intention to complete the procedure in two stages enables the periosteal layer to be closed with 5/0 polyglycolic acid and the skin to be closed with 6/0 nylon (**8.25–8.26**).

The second-stage procedure at about 4–6 months uses the same incision. The intention, after confirming that osseointegration has occurred, is to remove all of the soft tissue between periosteum and skin for approximately 2 cm around each fixture. The skin cuff around each protruding abutment will thus be tightly bound down and resists local irritation by skin movement (**8.27, 8.28**).

A small aperture is trephined in the thinned skin and a healing cap placed on the protruding abutment to hold a half-inch ribbon gauze soaked in Proflavine and keep the skin close to periosteum. This is changed at five days and removed at 10 days. The abutment is ready for impression taking at about three weeks (**8.29**).

Currently, the installation and attachments of abutments is being completed in one stage and works well. It is, however, reserved for adults and rigid fixation of the implants placed. Patients with craniofacial distortion often have abnormal amounts of bone, and caution about completing both stages at the same time should be exercised in these cases.

Unsightly auricular remnants require careful evaluation before removal is advised. Sometimes an emotional attachment to a previous unpleasant mass requires careful guidance for the patient before the second stage.

At the surgical operation to position the abutments, the skin is reduced to a 1–1.5 mm thickness over a radius of 1.0 cm around them. The cuffs will then be allowed to heal completely. It is likely in most cases with congenital defects of the ear that developmental remnants will also have been removed. Where possible a tragus is preserved or created by plastic surgery.

Prosthetic technique

A special tray may be prepared from a simple alginate impression of the face, or the surgical template may make a suitable tray when modified, to accept the passage of transfer impression copings attached to the abutments. It is important to ensure that each abutment protrudes 1.5–2 mm above the surface of the skin in order to provide proper clearance of the prosthesis from the face. The impression must be recorded in a polymer which is relatively rigid when set, creating an accurate record of the relationships of the implant abutments (**8.30**).

The use of a wash impression within a closely fitted tray produces a suitable amount of displacement of the tissue so that the anterior margin of the prosthesis can be closely applied as a knife-edge fit against the skin. Prior to making the impression, it is helpful to mark the skin with the orientation marks of facial landmarks or reference planes. These then transfer onto the cast and assist the technician in orientating the trial ear correctly. Also, it is necessary to apply petroleum jelly to the hair on the impression site, having pinned most locks out of the way.

The impression is removed and replica abutments are screwed to the impression copings before the impression is cast in stone.

The wax trial ear prosthesis may now be adapted to the cast and then checked for position upon the patient by removing the healing caps and fitting it over the abutments.

The construction of the prosthesis is now carried out in two steps. First, a round or oval gold alloy bar

(2 mm diameter) is positioned and soldered to gold alloy cylinders secured to the dummy abutments (**8.31**). The undersurface of the bar is separated by 3–4 mm from the cast. Cantilever extensions to the bar project in directions that will provide sites of anchorage that prevent rotation of the prosthesis around a fulcrum between the abutments. A zone around the bar is now blocked out with Plaster of Paris so that an acrylic resin substructure may be formed which encloses the sleeves or retaining clips positioned upon the bar. Secondly, the wax trial ear is modified to fit over the substructure before it is invested in a three-part mould. Various silicone elastomers (e.g. Silastic, Cosmesil) which cure at room temperature are available for manufacturing the prosthesis. Good colour-matching, high tear-resistance and dimensional stability characterise their performance.

The mould is packed in the presence of the patient so that pigments may be incorporated into the silicone polymer in order to achieve close representation of the skin tones. To ensure adherence of the elastomer to the acrylic resin substructure this is lightly roughened and cleaned with acetone before a primer is applied (**8.32**).

Retention of the ear prosthesis upon the bar should be checked (**8.33**). The patient must be instructed to place and remove it. Since the bar may not be readily seen by the patient, advice should also be given to a companion of the patient on cleansing the abutments and the surrounding cuffs. A bactericidal soap is beneficial in keeping the skin healthy (**8.34, 8.35**).

Monitoring of the effectiveness of the prosthesis is necessary at frequent visits initially and then, after one year, at periods of six to 12 months. Although the prosthesis is vented and made free of contact with the face except at its anterior leading edge, the cutaneous cuffs may become hyperaemic and bleed unless a good standard of hygiene is achieved. This problem is usually resolved rapidly with topical application of an antifungal, antibacterial steroidal cream, e.g. Terra-Cortril ointment.

Production of an orbital facial prosthesis

Where the orbital cavity has been exenterated and the patient remains free of recurrence of the tumour, it may be appropriate to use an implant-stabilised prosthesis. This incorporates an artificial globe and is clipped to skull implants in the superior and lateral margins of the bony orbit. If the prosthesis is separate and free from an oral obturator so that it is undisturbed by masticatory loading, then it may be retained by magnets. These are mounted in the prosthesis and link to the keepers which are usually screwed individually into each abutment.

Linking the abutments with a round gold alloy bar soldered to cylinders screwed to the abutments may be possible only when two or three implants angled at less than 30° to each other are used. Greater divergence and larger numbers of implants hinder the path of insertion of the cylinders upon the abutments.

Careful clinical appraisal of the orbital cavity is required to ensure that sufficient depth exists to accommodate the prosthesis and implants. It is important to be certain that the globe and pupil can be matched with the natural remaining eye for prominence and level, respectively. Palpation of the orbital rim should reveal any sites of discontinuity and defects. Facial contours should also be inspected to identify the potential site of the margin of the prosthesis, which should ideally lie in the skin folds in order to disguise the border. The colours of the iris and the sclera should be matched to available artificial eyes. Also the shape and extent of the eyebrows and eyelashes should be observed so that important facial features are represented in the final prosthesis. Where possible the eyebrow on the defective side should be preserved.

An impression of the entire face anterior to the ears and extending from the forehead to the chin is next recorded in an elastic material (**8.36**). A rubber strap, draught-excluding strip or cardboard strip is adapted to the face. A seal may be made against the cardboard with damp paper or wet cottonwool in order to contain the fluid mix of alginate impression material. This is backed with Plaster of Paris before the impression is withdrawn and a cast poured (**8.37**). The defective site is marked by the maxillo-facial technician to show the horizontal level and central position for the pupil, matching the normal side of the face. A wax base is laid down and cut to the proposed border. A carefully chosen pre-made artificial globe is set in position and the remaining contours created by carving and moulding wax to form a trial prosthesis (**8.38**). This is first examined for correct form when positioned upon the face. It is particularly important for the surgeon to assess the correct location and angulation for each proposed implant so that there is no conflict between the expected surface shape and the retaining elements on the abutments. For this reason it may be decided to use specially developed magnets or precision attachments with a low profile (e.g. Rotherman) rather than a bar.

The planning is completed with suitable X-rays, e.g. postero-anterior and lateral skull projections recorded in a cephlostat together with a CT scan. The surgeon is then able to confirm his choice of sites for the skull fixtures, marking them upon the study cast. The surgical procedure follows the same steps as described for the ear (**8.39**). It is important to separate the fixtures by at least 15 mm. Likewise, when the abutments are connected, they should ultimately protrude 2 mm from the skin surface. A sufficient number of implants should be positioned to allow for failure of osseointegration which commonly exceeds other sites in the skull, especially in consequence of the effect of previous irradiation. Specially made small screwdrivers and other surgical instruments may be needed because of the restriction of access in the socket.

In view of the opposing positions of the abutments, it may be necessary to record two working impressions with transfer impression copings located on a group of abutments, e.g. those in the supra-orbital ridge.

The maxillo-facial technician may then decide if two separate bars are united or left isolated with, for example, one below the supra-orbital ridge and another medial to the lateral socket margin.

The prosthesis is constructed in a manner similar to one replacing an ear, i.e. with a transparent margin (**8.40, 8.41, 8.42**). Venting is important to avoid moisture condensation below the prosthesis. These vents may be sited in the eyelid to hide the orifices (**8.43**).

Production of a nasal or facial prosthesis

Surgical excision or traumatic loss of the nose may extend to adjacent areas of the face. Where possible it is highly desirable to maintain continuity of the lips in order to permit closure of the circumoral aperture.

Clinical examination should identify the position of the margins of the prosthesis on the face and the relation with the oral tissues. For example, loss of the anterior part of the palate and dental arch may offer sites into which to position oral implants. Other key areas for inserting skull implants are the glabella and root of the zygoma. A plan is required to create well-bound-down skin or mucosa surrounding the fixture abutments.

A study cast prepared from a full-face impression, together with profile and frontal portrait photographs, will assist in the subsequent modelling of a trial prosthesis.

Inspection of the CT scan should confirm the suitability of available bone. It is then possible to devise an individual frame that can provide the retentive mechanism and support for the prosthesis. Ideally the frame should be constructed in one piece by soldering bars to cylinders that fit the abutments or to specially constructed components built around the cylinders. An acrylic substructure containing retentive clips is needed as a foundation for the silicone prosthesis (**8.44, 8.45**).

The prosthesis should be closely adapted at the margins and have apertures in the site of the anterior nares to allow respiration through the nasal cavity. At the inferior surface it may be necessary to create inner and outer contacts to avoid seeping of oral or nasal fluids.

Combination prostheses restoring both intra-oral and extra-oral defects require maximum use of available anchorage and the preservation of areas important to the support and function of the prosthesis. For example, preservation of the posterior hard palate and tuberosity offer sites for implant insertion and significantly contribute to effective swallowing by maintaining a firm contact with the prosthesis and the necessary attachment for soft palate function.

Very careful planning is required to ensure that the patient is able to insert the prosthesis comfortably and to withdraw it without damage. Proper supervision of home care is needed to be certain of effective cleaning of the abutment sites and to check for evidence of chronic inflammation or infection of the tissues of the epithelial cuffs. This requires a regular recall procedure. Changes in the colour of the extra-oral prosthesis due to exposure to industrial atmospheres, including smoke, and sunlight may then be corrected by retinting or remaking the prosthesis. Inspection of those tissues having reduced sensation is especially important to confirm that the traumatic effects of wearing the prosthesis do not go unnoticed, as these can otherwise produce dramatic improvements in the daily life of the patient.

169

SUMMARY OF TREATMENT PLANNING REQUIREMENTS AND DECISIONS BY TEAM FOR SELECTED CASES

Information required

1: Clinical appraisal of defective tissue area

- Estimation of likely retention and support sites from implants.
- Consideration of surface contours to identify redundant tissue and penetration by the abutments of unfavourable skin or mucosa.
- Determination of desirable form and border shape of prosthesis.

2: Radiographic examination

- CT scan to determine suitable sites of available bone.

3: Laboratory assessment

- Diagnostic model for preparation of trial prosthesis.
- Template for locating implant sites.
- Preliminary prosthesis design.

4: Decisions taken

- Surgical stage 1: Implantation
  Decision on number, type, position, angulation and relationships of fixtures.
- Surgical stage 2: Abutment connection
  Penetration of skin: decision on thickness, movable or fixed cuff, hair-free or grafted skin.
  Penetration of mucosa: decision on thickness and fixed or mobile cuff, having non-keratinised mucosa; need for mucosal graft.

5: Prosthesis construction

- Determination of perimeter identified by fixed or mobile tissue and tissue contour.
- Retention mechanism: separate or linked abutments using bar, magnets or precision attachments.
- Ventilation.
- Additional characterisation (eyebrows, moustache, hairstyle, spectacles).

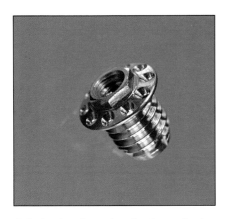

8.1 A titanium implant made by Nobelpharma for use in the skull. The area of contact with bone is enhanced by the flange that compensates for the short length of fixture.

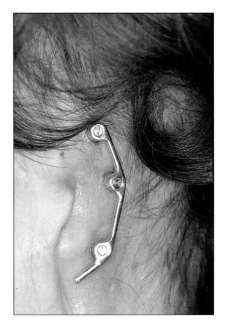

8.2 The superstructure screwed to the implant abutments to provide anchorage for the artificial ear.

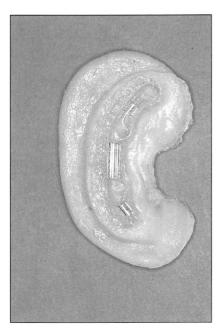

8.3 The fit surface of the prosthesis incorporating retaining clips which engage the bar.

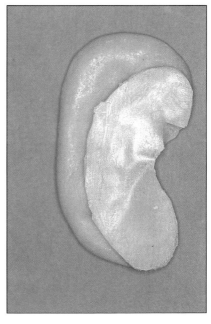

8.4 Use of adhesive tape with a previous prosthesis.

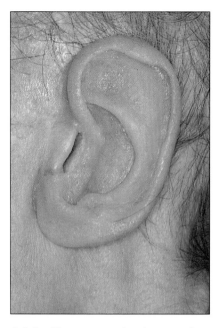

8.5 A silicone prosthesis restoring an ear lost traumatically in a road traffic accident.

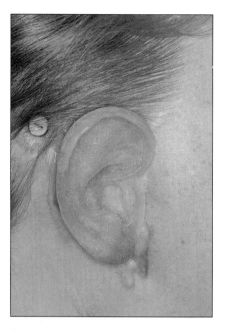

8.6 A hearing aid abutment is located behind the trial artificial ear.

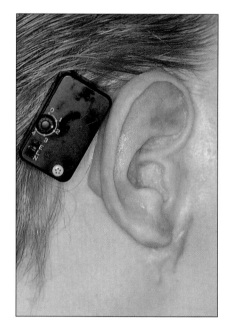

8.7 The bone-anchored hearing aid is positioned within the hairline and clear of contact with the prosthetic helix.

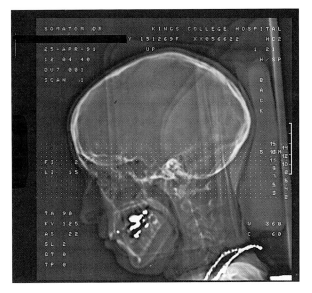 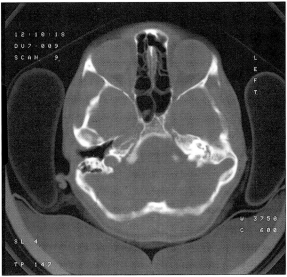

8.8a CT (CAT) scan at the level of the mastoid process of the skull. 8.8b Reformatted image as an axial slice showing contrasting thicknesses of the mastoid bones. The defective left external ear can also be seen.

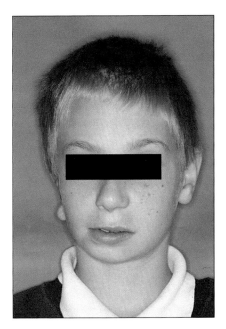

8.9 A patient with craniofacial microsomia demonstrating an abnormal position of the ear lobe. Facial asymmetry is a common problem.

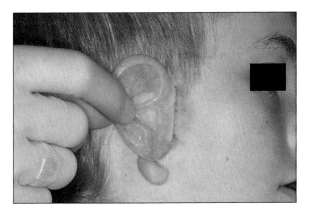

8.10 Localising a trial prosthesis behind the mobile skin overlying the condyle.

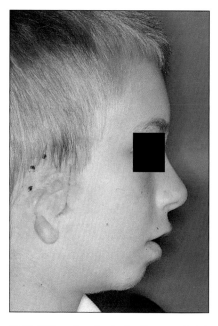

8.11 Siting implants in the mastoid below the bulk of the anthelix within the perimeter of the ear.

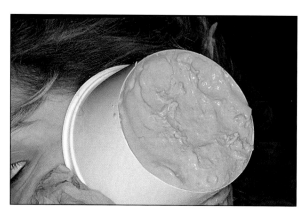

8.12 Recording a primary impression of the defective side of the face with a 2:1 water to powder mix of alginate material.

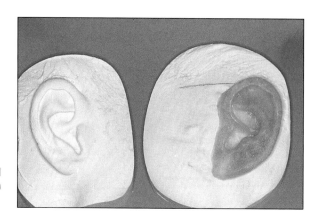

8.13 Casts poured from impressions of the left and right side of the face. A hand-carved wax ear has been prepared by the maxillo-facial technician.

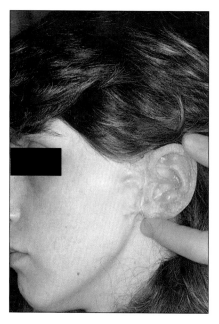

8.14 Siting the trial prosthesis on another patient.

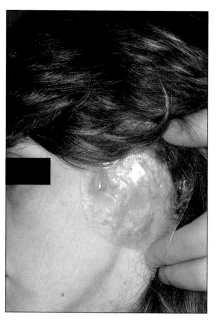

8.15 Positioning the template on the face in order to indicate the preferred implant sites.

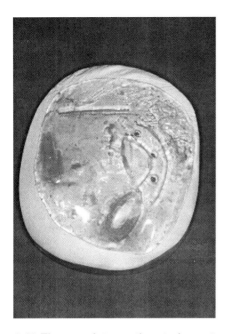

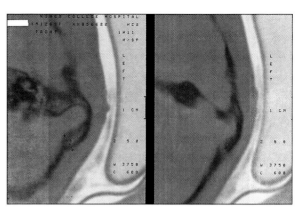

8.17 Reformatted images contrasting the available thicknesses of bone at different positions on the affected side.

8.16 The template on the study cast is marked with a reference line to the tail of the eyebrow, three possible implant sites and the perimeter of the ear.

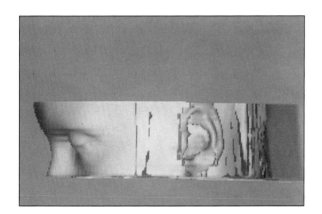

8.18 A computer image derived from the CT scan. A mirror image of the normal ear has been transposed to the defective side of the face to assist in assessment of the possible result of treatment.

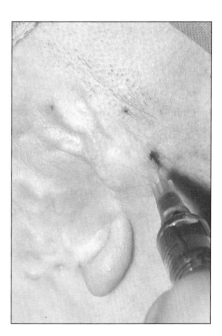

8.19 Marking through the skin to the surface of the skull at the chosen sites indicated by the prior application of the template.

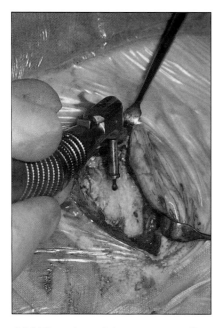

8.20 Elevation of the cutaneous flap to expose the mastoid and enable penetration of bone with a rose-head bur at the marked site.

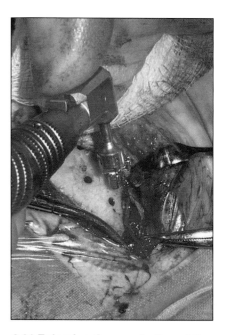

8.21 Enlarging the penetration of the skull with a counter-sink bur in order to create sufficient depth for the implant flange.

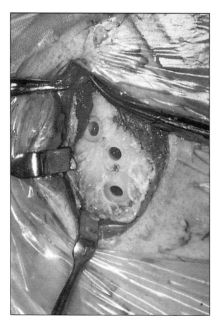

8.22 Completed preparation of the bony canals to receive the skull fixtures.

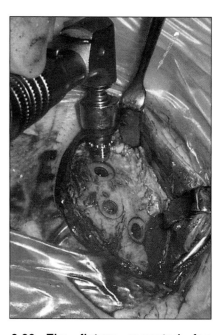

8.23 The fixture mounted for insertion in the canal.

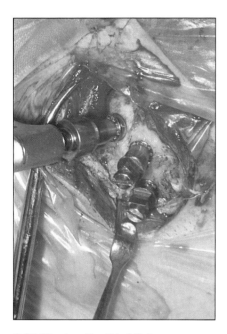

8.24 Placing the third fixture.

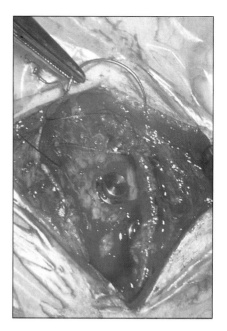

8.25 The mounts have been removed and cover screws placed prior to wound closure.

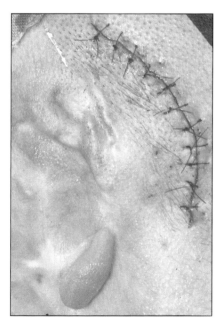

8.26 Completed operation showing a suture line remote from the implants.

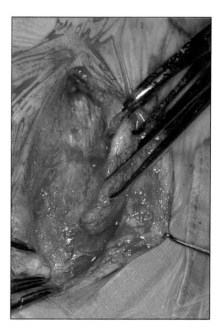

8.27 The essential step of thinning the skin during the second-stage operation. This ensures a tight thin non-mobile cutaneous cuff around the abutment.

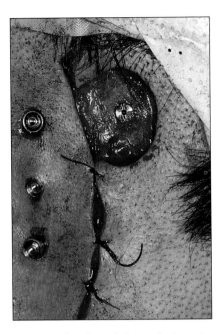

8.28 Application of three abutments for use with prosthesis together with a remote abutment for the bone-anchored hearing aid. Note: the hair-bearing skin has been excised and a free graft applied.

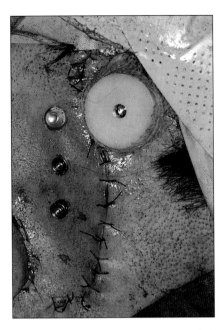

8.29 The addition of a special healing cap with a ribbon gauze pack to obtain close apposition of the graft against the tissue bed.

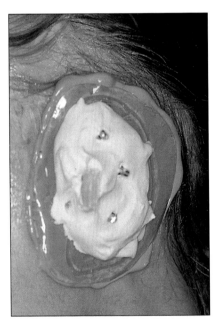

8.30 A special tray impression recorded over the abutments using Plaster of Paris to stabilise the transfer copings.

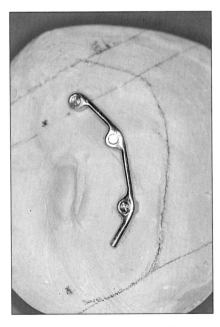

8.31 The master cast carrying the cylinders and soldered bar upon dummy abutments.

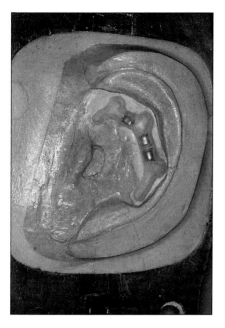

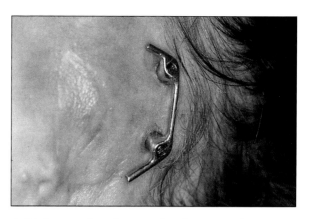

8.33 A completed case showing two abutments carrying the bar.

8.32 A laboratory mould prepared for packing silicone elastomer onto the prepared acrylic cover incorporating retaining clips.

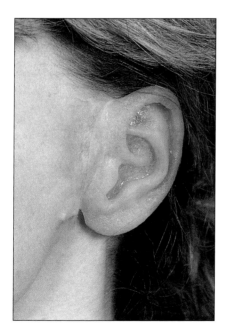

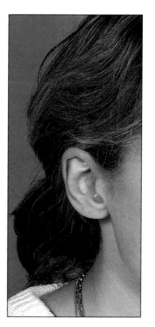
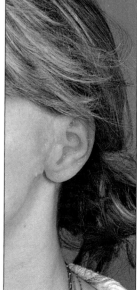

8.34 The prosthesis clipped in position.

8.35 Normal right ear (left) and prosthetic left ear (right).

179

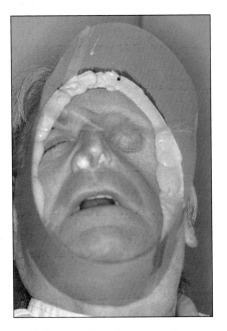

8.36 Preparation for recording an impression of most of the face.

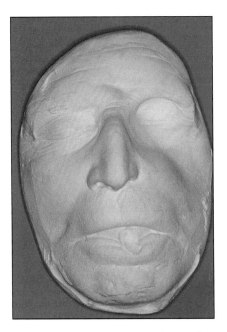

8.37 Study cast poured to the impression, identifying the defect.

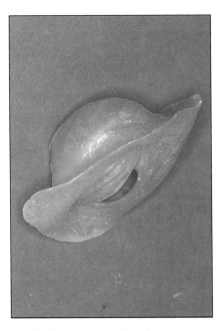

8.38 Trial wax prosthesis showing necessary depth to accommodate the orbital prosthesis and retaining elements.

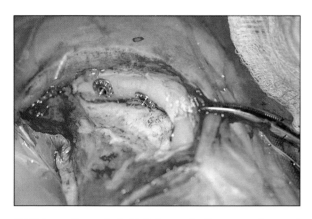

8.39 Location of skull fixtures in the superior and lateral aspects of the orbital rim.

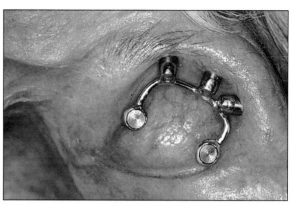

8.40 Abutments carrying three cylinders and a bar incorporating magnets.

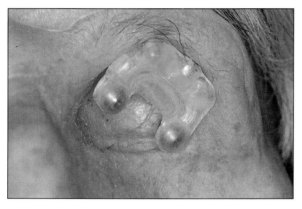

8.41 Acrylic shell incorporating clips and magnetic keepers.

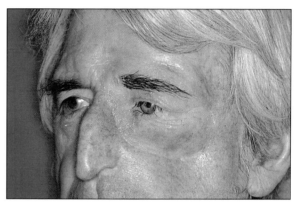

8.42 The prosthesis in position.

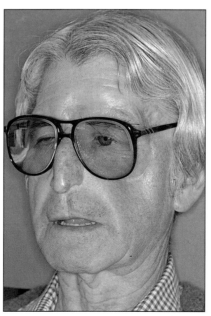

8.43 Spectacles may be used to camouflage the margins of the prosthesis.

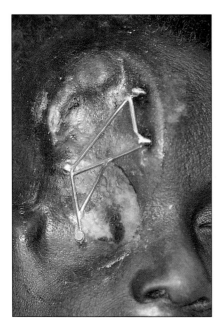

8.44 Use of a linked frame to stabilise an extensive facial prosthesis and distribute the loads widely.

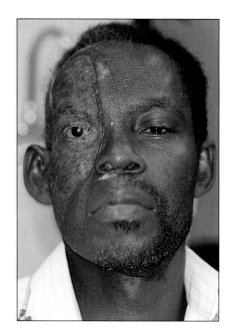

8.45 Facial prosthesis *in situ*.

9. Problems

Introduction

The inherently complex nature of implant treatment makes it more prone to problems than more simple procedures. While prevention is preferable to a cure, difficulties cannot always be avoided. When they arise, symptomatic treatment must be preceded by identification and, where possible, removal of the cause.

Whilst some problems are very specific in their nature and cause, others are more varied in presentation. These often originate in decisions taken long before implant insertion or reflect poor surgical or prosthetic technique. Their causes may be less readily identified and they can be conveniently considered separately from those with a more specific presentation.

Difficulties which arise in the period immediately following implant insertion can often be traced to incomplete diagnosis, or lack of care with treatment or infection control. Problems that occur later tend to reflect failure of materials or, sometimes, the tissue–implant interface.

Informed consent

Whilst informed consent to treatment is essential on legal and ethical grounds, care provided for well-informed patients who are effective partners in their own treatment is more likely to be successful. Advice must be provided by the dentist, but the level of detail which it is appropriate to provide for a patient is a matter for clinical judgement. For example, the person receiving conventional complete dentures for the first time would expect more information than the seasoned denture wearer.

In the field of implant treatment, patients' knowledge is usually scanty and often coloured by a belief in the ability of the procedure to overcome many oral problems. Some do genuinely consider that they will receive a completely maintenance-free analogue of the natural dentition, which will be *in situ* when they recover from the first surgical stage. When instead they are provided with an overdenture over a more protracted period, with intervals when a prosthesis cannot be worn, not surprisingly difficulties ensue.

Because treatment with implants is predominantly a team activity, confusion can arise if the responsibilities of the team members are not defined from the start. Key issues which must be addressed are:

- What is the nature of the patient's problem?
- What are the treatment alternatives and why has implant therapy been recommended?
- Why has a particular implant system been selected?
- What type of prosthesis is to be employed?
- What types of failure of the prosthesis might occur and how would they be handled?
- How many implants are to be inserted?
- What clinical procedures will be carried out and what will be their effect; for example, the inability to use a denture for one or two weeks?
- What is the probability of failure of integration and what will happen if it occurs? Will implants be removed, could they be replaced and who would be responsible for the work and its costs? Patients must be informed that, even with meticulous care, integration cannot be guaranteed.
- If it is not found possible at surgery to carry out the procedure as envisaged, what might happen and what would be the implications for treatment? In the worst situation, implant treatment might have to be abandoned; more commonly it is found that fewer implants can be inserted, necessitating the use of a removable prosthesis.
- What is the patient's role in maintenance of the implants?
- What long-term servicing might be required and when?

Failure to establish the ground rules before starting any treatment is always unwise; in complex and expensive procedures it is foolhardy and can lead to considerable problems.

General problems

Many of the problems under this heading reflect problems of patient selection and are dealt with in more detail in Chapter 4.

Case selection

The selection of patients who will benefit significantly from implant treatment is one of the more difficult and challenging aspects of this type of therapy. It is important that it is handled thoroughly. Among the factors to be considered are:

Systemic factors

- **Psychological problems.** Some patients who seek treatment with implants suffer from psychological disorders which may contraindicate the use of fixtures.
- **Drug abuse.** Patients who are habitual drug abusers are unsuitable candidates for implant treatment.
- **Ability to cooperate.** It is axiomatic that a patient for whom implant treatment is proposed should be able to collaborate with both the surgical and prosthodontic procedures and the subsequent home maintenance.
- **Ability to provide appropriate oral hygiene.** Dental implant superstructures rapidly become coated with plaque and calculus if they are not kept thoroughly clean. Failure to maintain high levels of oral hygiene can lead to breakdown of the tissues around the implants and their ultimate failure.
- **Systemic disease influencing integration.** Patients who suffer from disorders of bone metabolism such as osteoporosis may not readily produce an osseointegrated implant interface and medical advice should be sought as to the severity of their condition.
- **Systemic disease predisposing to infection.** These conditions, such as poorly controlled diabetes mellitus, prejudice the success of implant treatment.
- **Smoking.** Tobacco smoking is associated with increased failure of implant treatment.

Local factors

- **Implant-centred treatment.** Problems may arise if treatment is based solely on its advantages, without due consideration of the patient's dental needs, both immediately and in the long term.
- **Insertion and restorative problems.** Problems may arise if due allowance has not been made for the need to be able both to insert and to restore the planned implants.
- **Functional problems.** The planned prostheses should have the potential to meet the patient's needs without producing unacceptable new problems.

Surgical problems

Bone assessment

The quantity, shape and quality of the bone into which dental implants are inserted will have a profound effect on the subsequent treatment. Inadequate quantity will result in implants which project beyond the bone surface. A small protrusion may eventfully become covered with bone where it lifts the periosteum, a more extensive one will not.

The shape of the ridge determines the orientation of the implants if they are to be contained within it. If this is unfavourable then the implants my be inappropriately positioned or angled, making restoration difficult.

Implants which are placed in bone which has a low density with a thin cortex and few trabeculae are less likely to integrate. This and other causes of failure to integrate are considered below.

Soft-tissue problems

The principal difficulty which can arise in connection with soft tissues is the placing of implants too close to mobile tissues. This is often seen in the anterior aspect of the mandible (**9.13**) where fixtures are placed too far lingually so that the superstructure traumatises the floor of the mouth.

Problems can also arise if the fixtures are placed in areas where the submucosa is very thick. This can cause difficulties in accommodating the superstructure and abutments and the cuff may be more prone to infection. Soft-tissue resection at the time of implant placement can minimise this problem.

Damage to adjacent structures

The placing of dental implants in severely resorbed jaws brings with it an increased risk of damage to adjacent structures. Some will subsequently heal, many will suffer irreversible damage. Those which are particularly prone to involvement include the floor of the mouth, the mandibular canal, the mental neuro-vascular bundle, the roots of adjacent teeth, and the nose and antra. Damage to teeth and nerves is usually irreversible, whereas other structures may heal given appropriate management.

Wound breakdown

Breakdown of the wound over an implant may reflect failure to relieve adequately any temporary prosthesis where it covers the implant, or inappropriate flap design. Where breakdown occurs some time after implant insertion then it may cause few problems, as it essentially represents slightly premature exposure of the fixture. More serious is exposure in the first few weeks after implant insertion when the risk of subsequent failure of integration is considerable. In these circumstances, the wound should be thoroughly debrided, the cover screw replaced with a new one and soft tissue cover re-established.

Prosthodontic problems

Prosthesis design

Three groups of errors may be recognised: functional, hygiene-related and overloading.

Functional problems relate to the appearance of the prosthesis, the patient's ability to masticate and speak when using it. All are considered in detail below.

Failure to design the prosthesis so that the patient can maintain good oral hygiene is a common cause of problems which are often design-related.

The effects of overloading can occur in either the superstructure or the implant–host interface. Both can have severe consequences, although the former is more easily rectified. They usually result from failure to follow recommended guidelines as to the number and length of implants to be used in a particular configuration, or the degree of cantilevering which it is appropriate to employ. They may also be seen in patients who have patterns of parafunctional occlusal activity.

Poor construction

Poorly constructed implant superstructures inevitably predispose to subsequent clinical failure.

Infection

Infection in the region of the implant site can arise at any time after implant insertion, but is more common in the period immediately afterwards. It can result in either acute or chronic inflammation, and its major significance relates to its influence on osseointegration. The management of the infection itself should follow normal procedures and be aimed at bringing the infection under control as rapidly as possible. Methods will often include the use of hot salt mouth washes and chlorhexidine mouthwashes, accompanied by systemic measures where appropriate.

Infection of the implant site immediately after insertion may arise because of poor surgical technique or inadequate home care. It is identified by the classical signs and symptoms of inflammation and should be treated immediately and thoroughly. However, it usually results in failure of integration.

More superficial infections can occur in the suture line and are less hazardous where this lies some distance from the fixture. They may arise around retained sutures and usually respond well to their removal and local palliative measures.

The risk of infection falls after the removal of the sutures and then rises again after the second surgical stage.

Systemic disorders that slow the healing process or reduce the effectiveness of the inflammatory and healing mechanisms may also be associated with peri-implant infection, of which diabetes mellitus is a classic example.

Failure to integrate

This problem is usually diagnosed radiographically, unless the implant has been connected to the oral cavity and breakdown of the interface with bone has proceeded to the level where the implant is loose. Whilst integration has been defined by some workers, there is less certainty as to the extent of the integrated interface which is necessary for success. Traditional clinical methods of assessing mobility are of no value other than to recognise loss of integration, and recourse is currently made to radiographic analysis.

The radiographic appearances of integration are of the presence of a layer of bone next to the implant surface and minimal cratering of the ridge crest where it is penetrated by the implant (**9.7, 9.8**). Where there is evidence of reduced bone density beside the implant, or apparently a space between the two, then integration must be suspect. It should be remembered, however, that a radiograph will portray only a very small section of the implant–host interface and that its resolution of detail is limited. Whilst serial radiographic evidence of change around an implant over a period of time is of considerable significance, a single view is rarely of as much value and clinical findings are the ultimate arbiters. Non-invasive techniques for assessing implant integration, including the use of resonance measurements, are currently under investigation and may, in the future, provide a better understanding of the phenomenon and its detection.

The systemic causes of failure of the integration process are usually associated with conditions in which bone metabolism is impaired, such as osteoporosis. Local factors include infection at the time of implant insertion, inappropriate surgical preparation of the bone by overheating, implant insertion in bone of unsuitable quality or inadequate initial fixation of the implant. Bone quality has been discussed in case assessment and it should be remembered that prior radiotherapy will reduce the healing capability of the tissue. Inadequate fixation has been shown to influence the quality of integration and reflect the initial fit of the implant. It can also be a problem where implants penetrate a covering epithelium *ab initio* and are thus potentially subject to external loads whilst healing occurs.

Where an implant which penetrates the mucosa from the time of insertion has been used, then it may reflect epithelial down-growth or the application of excessive loads to the implant during the initial healing period.

Implants which have failed to integrate should be removed and the region left to heal for 6–12 months, when a further fixture may be placed if necessary. Alternatively, a different site may be chosen or a 'sleeping' fixture brought into use. Commonly this will involve construction of a new prosthesis, modification of an existing one or the use of a temporary removable prosthesis in preference to a fixed implant bridge.

The failure of integration is most common in the first two years after the prosthesis is loaded. This may reflect overloading of poorly supported fixtures, for example 7 mm devices in the maxilla, or a pathological change in the patient, such as the onset of osteoporosis.

Fixture location

Problems arise on occasions as a result of inappropriate location of one or more fixtures. Whilst careful planning and the use of a surgeon's template should prevent such occurrences, they can arise through error or unanticipated problems during surgery. The difficulty may come to light only after the second stage of surgery and its effects vary with the latitude the restorative dentist has in placing the superstructure. Where an overdenture is to be used, there may be greater latitude than with a fixed superstructure, although the denture space will place restrictions on what may be achieved. There is also more flexibility in the lower jaw than in the upper and more flexibility in edentulous patients than in those who are to have a partially edentulous arch restored with a fixed superstructure. In these circumstances, the margin of error in the placing of the fixtures is very small as the positions of the superstructures are determined by the adjacent teeth. Implants placed too buccally will cause the superstructure to be too prominent, whilst those located too palatally will present the opposite problem, as well as impeding tongue movements in the lower jaw.

Whilst some situations are more flexible than others, all should be approached with a similar level of precision. Where implants are misplaced, a number of manoeuvres can be used to overcome the problem. Much will depend on the flexibility of the system employed. However, many include a variety of angled abutments which can be employed to correct misalignment with the dental arch. These may not provide as stable a linkage as a straight abutment and care should be taken if using them singly as occlusal loads tend to rotate them. They can, however, prevent the need to bring screws through the labial aspect of the prosthesis. As an alternative, some systems provide a tapered abutment which is intended for use with a single crown with its margin below the mucosa. This can be used in place of a standard abutment to permit some variation in location of the superstructure.

Where only one fixture is misplaced, consideration should be given to keeping it as a 'sleeper' and modifying the design accordingly. In more extreme situations it may be necessary to utilise a removable superstructure rather than a fixed one, as the greater freedom in design can often encompass the misplaced implants. In these situations, lack of space may, however, dictate the use of individual attachments with a low profile on each fixture.

Where gross misplacement has occurred, especially in critical applications, there may be no alternative but to remove the implants. The message of this problem is plain: design and plan the superstructure before placing the implants, anticipating how surgical problems may be overcome.

Pain

Pain is a rare complaint when using dental implants and has two principal causes associated with the implants themselves: looseness of an abutment and the creation of excessive stresses in the implant–patient system. It is also suggestive of failure of osseointegration if it occurs when tightening the screws which link the various components. In addition, discomfort can arise from the use of a removable prosthesis as with any other type of overdenture.

When an abutment does not fit precisely on a fixture then a patient often experiences considerable pain. This is usually sharp in nature and is due to pinching of the soft tissues between the two components and is relieved by tightening the fixing screw. Before this is done, the soft tissues may need to be infiltrated with a local anaesthetic and the cuff around the abutment retracted by gently running a pocket measuring probe in the crevice around the abutment. Problems can also arise where bone which has grown over the cover screw has not been completely cleared from the end of the fixture. As a result the abutment may not seat fully.

As the top of the fixture is usually 'sub-gingival', positioning the abutment by direct vision is not possible. As a result, problems often arise due to failure to relate accurately the fixture and the abutment when placing the latter. This may be especially difficult if these incorporate anti-rotation features which make their accurate assembly more difficult.

A check for the fit may be carried out radiographically or mechanically. Radiographs are of value only when they are at right angles to the long axis of the implant, and should be used sparingly for safety reasons. Where a hexagonal coupling is employed then the abutment should be grasped with a pair of forceps, the fixing screw gently loosened and an attempt made to rotate the abutment carefully backwards and forwards. If the two components are correctly related then this is not possible other than within the tolerance of the coupling, whilst incorrect seating is immediately evident by the ease with which further rotation is possible. Once the components are correctly aligned, the screw may be tightened.

Stresses in the implant system can arise as a result of an ill-fitting superstructure or excessive functional jaw deformation where a patient has a rigid prosthesis. Whilst the pain associated with a loose abutment is very sharp, stress-related pain is usually described as a dull ache or a feeling of pressure or clamping. Where it is caused by a poor fit of the superstructure then it is associated with its placement, whilst difficulties with jaw deformation are usually found with large frameworks and thinner mandibles.

Relief usually occurs when the superstructure is removed. A poor fit may not be immediately evident as the superstructure may fit only on one side of an abutment and must therefore be checked from all sides. Both this deficiency and one which is continuous around the abutment will produce forces on the implant when the screws retaining a linked superstructure are tightened. Deformation-related discomfort is less common but straightforward to diagnose, although its management may involve remaking the prosthesis with a precision attachment in the mid-line to allow a small amount of movement. It must be stressed that absence of discomfort is never evidence of a satisfactory fit.

Soft-tissue problems

Enlargement

Swelling of the soft tissues next to an implant is most commonly associated with looseness of an abutment and can be dramatic in its extent. It is not always painful. Fortunately, it resolves rapidly following correction of the fault (**9.4, 9.5**).

Soreness of the cuff around an abutment is observed in some patients, usually where the newly placed abutment penetrates mobile mucosa. If this prevents the patient cleaning the abutments effectively then oedema may ensue.

Another cause of this problem is impaction of food particles, such as poppy seeds, in the crevice between the abutment and the soft tissues. Such particles can often be washed out by gently irrigating the area with chlorhexidine solution using a fine-tipped disposable syringe. Care must be taken not to build up any pressure in the tissues. If this does not resolve the problem then it will be necessary to remove the abutment temporarily to gain access to the site.

The soft tissues related to the implant superstructure may also enlarge, and two situations can be recognised. One involves the spaces below a fixed superstructure, and the other is associated with relative movement of soft tissues and prosthesis. The first is sometimes observed below the retaining bars of overdentures and can obliterate the space between the bar and the ridge crest (**9.19**). The tissue is usually firm and not inflamed. A similar phenomenon is seen under the relief chambers in complete dentures. Some workers consider that the condition is also associated with poor oral hygiene.

The condition does not require correction if the tissues are not inflamed and cleaning of the implants is not impeded. Overgrowth can often be controlled mechanically by use of thick floss below the bar. Where a superadded inflammation is present, then the cause of this should be removed.

Mechanical irritation of the soft tissues by an overextended denture can give rise to a denture-related granuloma, the cause and management of which is the same as for a denture which is not implant-stabilised. An analogous situation arises where fixed prostheses are in contact with mobile tissue. This is sometimes observed where the lingual placing of a mandibular implant has resulted in the superstructure encroaching on the floor of the mouth (**9.20**). The region over the insertion of the genial muscles can be especially troublesome as this is often very prominent following alveolar resorption. The difficulty may sometimes be overcome by careful contouring of the superstructure to remove sharp edges, but in recalcitrant cases may require remaking the prosthesis. Care at the treatment planning stage, the construction of a diagnostic appliance and the preparation and use of a surgeon's template can often prevent this vexatious problem.

Fractured components

Endosseous implants are employed to transmit occlusal loads to the facial skeleton via a relatively rigid interface. They do so through mechanically complex systems which often incorporate a variety of components linked by small fixing devices. Applied loads are not known in any given clinical situation and superstructures are custom-fabricated by hand. Not surprisingly, such systems are prone to mechanical failure. The effects of this can vary from a minor irritation to a major clinical problem.

Failure of components may arise as a result of poor construction by the manufacturer, over-loading during assembly or overload during function.

The quality control of reputable manufacturers is such as to make component failure from this cause a rare event. Where components are supplied with batch or serial numbers, these should form part of the clinical record. They may be essential when matching replacement components or identifying potential failures associated with a particular production run.

Overloading during assembly is particularly likely with screws which can be over-tightened, leading to plastic deformation, thread deformation or stripping, and fracture. Under-tightening of screws may also be hazardous as this can allow excessive displacement of the components. Where screws have been removed and replaced several times they should be checked individually for thread damage.

Excessive loading by oral forces is most likely to occur where an implant superstructure is cantilevered either distally or buccally. This is because of the leverage effects which result (**9.16, 9.26**). A superstructure supported at each end cannot transmit forces to the fixtures larger than those which are applied. Cantilevering can result in loads several times greater than the applied force, after the fashion of a bottle opener.

The two groups of components most prone to failure are the various screws which many systems use and the superstructure itself. Management of the problem is inevitably dominated by its correction. This must not be at the expense of identifying and eradicating its cause.

Screw failure

Screws may cause problems through fracture, damage to the head or stripping of the thread. Fracture is most likely to occur through excessive occlusal loads or over-tightening by hand, which is largely prevented by using mechanical torque-controlled screwdrivers.

The identification of a fractured screw varies with its function. If it is the sole method of securing a superstructure then the event will be immediately evident. If it is one of a series of retainers then the fracture may become evident only during routine removal of the prosthesis, or occasionally in a radiographic examination. The continued use of a fixed prosthesis where screws are fractured may result in distortion or fracture of the superstructure or loss of osseointegration.

The management of the failure usually involves removal of the remaining part of the screw and its replacement with a new component. Difficulties arise if this has broken off within its housing or it lies below the orifice of the mucosal cuff, making access problematical. In these circumstances, infiltration with a local anaesthetic containing a vaso-constrictor can aid access and control pain. If the end of the screw can be grasped with a pair of fine mosquito forceps then removal is easy. If not, then the screw can usually be gently unwound by placing a sharp probe on its end and rotating the tip around the long axis of the screw. Attempts to use rotary instruments to remove screws only bur over the edges of the components and make removal more difficult. Should the screw fail to respond to attention with a probe then some manufacturers provide, often on a loan basis through their agents, a customised screw extractor.

Damaged screw heads can result from misuse of a screwdriver, although this can be difficult to avoid if access is restricted or the screws have been placed at a pronounced angle to the occlusal plane, especially if they are deep to the occlusal surface (**9.32**). The problem most often occurs as a result of applying full torque to the screwdriver when it is not fully seated or does not have its long axis coincident with that of the screw. This is more common when using a powered screwdriver, as inevitably some tactile feedback is lost, and finger-operated screwdrivers are to be preferred when initially adjusting awkwardly placed screws. Slotted screws are prone to burring over of the edges of the slot. Hexagonal heads can be rounded out internally by the gradual seating of a driver whilst it is rotating under load. This commonly occurs if the socket has not been fully cleared of debris before attempting removal.

The pattern of screw used should always be entered in the clinical records and the use of a silicone rubber seal will provide a further check on the type. This technique also obviates the problem of a temporary filling material becoming impacted in the socket. Screw heads can be irretrievably damaged by use of the wrong pattern or size of driver, particularly if this is driven mechanically. Powered drivers should be used only once the screw pattern and size have been positively identified and the operator is satisfied that the driver is fully seated.

Damaged slots can often be restored by deepening with a small bur However, once a hexagonal socket has been damaged the head usually has to be ground off the screw to allow disassembly of the components. As this makes the situation more difficult to manage, it should be employed only as a last resort. When doing this, care must be taken not to damage other parts of the implant.

Worn screw threads rarely present problems as they are evident when attempting to tighten the screw. A visual check confirms both the fault and the need to use a replacement.

Superstructure fracture

Implant superstructures are subjected to considerable loads from occlusal forces and, in the case of the lower jaw, to a lesser extent mandibular deformation. As the superstructure of a fixed prosthesis is curved to the form of the dental arch and may be cantilevered, it is often subject in function to twisting and bending moments. These may result in fracture of the prosthesis as a result of overload or fatigue failure. In the case of overdentures, the link between the prosthesis and the implants is by a coupling which will allow some movement, without which fracture would occur. As the two systems are prone to different types of failure, they may be considered separately.

Fixed superstructures. Fracture or bending of a cast superstructure is uncommon if care has been taken in its construction and the recommended dimensions used. Failure usually arises where loads are above average, as will arise with long cantilevers, opposing natural teeth, heavy occlusal loads, patients who grind their teeth and bridges which carry canine guidance. In the absence of an accurate method of predicting loads, the dentist should be cautious in these situations.

Faced with a fractured superstructure, the clinician will first need to maintain the patient's oral function. If the fracture is of a distal cantilever then the remaining superstructure can often continue to function in the interim period. Where the fracture is in the middle of a fixed superstructure then it will be necessary to carry out a temporary repair with wire and self- or light-cured resin. If this is not practicable then a temporary denture should be made if an old prosthesis cannot be modified to fill this role. Following identification of the cause of the fracture, a new superstructure should then be made.

Overdentures. Overdentures function by gaining stability from both the mucosa of the denture-bearing area and the implant fixtures. Because the mechanical characteristics of the two are very different, care must be taken to ensure that the distribution of loads between them is controlled. Most implant-stabilised overdentures are used with implants in the anterior part of the jaw and under vertical loads will thus tend to rotate around the fixtures. Some operators use a muco-displacing impression procedure to minimise relative displacement under load in these situations. Even when this technique is used, it should be combined with appropriate manoeuvres to control force distribution which involves both linear vertical movement and rotation. It is important that the attachments allow for this and that links permitting only linear movement are not utilised. In addition to allowing for rotation, space must be allowed for the relative linear movement of the two parts of the attachment under vertical loads. This is usually achieved with a spacer which is employed when locating the attachment in the denture. If this room is not provided then excessive forces will be placed on the attachments, causing fracture of the denture base, the implant superstructure or the attachments. This can arise as a result of alveolar resorption which allows the denture to 'sink' in relation to the implants.

If a bar type of attachment is employed then this may utilise distal cantilevers to reduce rotation of the denture away from the mucosa in the molar regions. These can become subject to heavy occlusal loads as a result of alveolar resorption or failure to use a spacer when locating the clips. This may result in fracture of the bar or gold cylinder (**9.26**) and cantilevers should not therefore normally be longer than 8 mm.

The rebasing of overdentures may be required to correct the effects of alveolar resorption or design and construction errors, and is described below.

Overdenture superstructures. Overdentures can be stabilised either with individual retainers mounted on each fixture or more commonly by a bar linking the implants. These may be cantilevered distally to reduce the rotation of the prosthesis. However, if these are too long then the cantilever may fracture. These breaks often run through the gold cylinder on the abutment. The patient can usually continue to use the denture but repair of the bar is often easier if the denture is used as a special tray, which then requires its removal from the patient for several days. The procedure involves rebasing the denture and relocating the attachments, and is described in the section on rebasing.

Fracture or loss of teeth. The causes of these are similar to those with tooth-retained prostheses and reflect poor bonding or excessive loading. The former is more likely to occur with acrylic teeth, if they are heavily cross-linked or have been contaminated with tinfoil substitute (cold mould seal) or wax. Porcelain teeth are retained solely by mechanical means. Excessive loading arises where liberties have been taken with the forces to which the teeth will be subjected.

Repairs can often be carried out at the chair side using standard techniques and self- or light-curing resin. The method does not produce as strong a result as a heat-cured repair, which must be carried out in the laboratory. If the failure was due to mechanical overload then it will recur unless the cause is identified and removed. It may be wise to evaluate the occlusion in the mouth, and to remount the prosthesis on an articulator.

Superstructure wear. One problem which may sometimes be encountered where patients use overdentures opposed by natural teeth is a tendency to grind the natural teeth against the implant superstructure when the denture is left out for hygiene reasons, for example at night. This can cause marked wear of the superstructures and may require the use of a night guard made in acrylic resin to protect the fixtures. This should have minimal mucosal coverage otherwise it defeats the object of leaving the denture out!

Functional problems

Air leakage

This complaint is most commonly associated with fixed superstructures and may arise with maxillary and mandibular prostheses, although it is more common with the former. It arises from the need to provide a space below the mucosal surface of the bridge to permit cleaning of the abutments and the superstructure in this region. As a result air and saliva may escape during speech. Patients should always be warned of this potential problem during treatment planning. With practice, many learn to overcome the difficulty, others are helped by the provision of a removable obturator made either in hard acrylic resin or silicone elastomer. In severe cases it may be necessary to replace the superstructure with one of a different design or even a removable prosthesis. Before replacement, diagnostic additions to the existing appliance may prove helpful.

Appearance

Whilst it could be argued that no prosthesis should be completed until the patient has given his or her approval of the trial appliance, sadly this does not totally obviate problems with subsequent dissatisfaction. Many of these are common to conventional prostheses. Where they involve changes in tooth shade then correction is relatively straightforward. Where more major alterations are requested then the possibilities for change are limited by the positions of the fixtures, the need to allow for oral hygiene and the superstructure design. If the abutments are not coincident with the teeth then they may need to be disguised with gumwork.

Lip trapping

Another problem which can arise relates to trapping of the lip above a fixed maxillary superstructure if the teeth have had to be cantilevered well in front of the ridge to allow for alveolar resorption. Careful extension of a flange, provided that the patient can maintain good hygiene, often controls this problem, although sometimes recourse may have to be made to a removable flange.

Some patients complain of being able to see the abutments and this occasionally arises due to under-extension of the superstructure towards the sulcus so that the abutments are seen in extreme movements of the lip. This should not be confused with the complaint by the patient that they can displace their lip far enough to see the abutments, which is essential to permit their cleaning!

Soft-tissue support

Complaints of lack of support for the soft tissues can arise in respect of both the lips and the cheeks. The former may be determined by the degree of cantilevering which it is possible to achieve, and the latter is inevitable with most fixed superstructures unless they can gain support from implants in the molar region. If it is intended to use a fixed superstructure then the trial denture which the patient uses to gain an impression of the final result should be trimmed to provide a reliable estimate of the support which will be provided by the final prosthesis. Once the appliances have been completed, there is little that can be done to correct matters without major changes. In some circumstances the only option may be to replace the fixed superstructure with a removable one which can provide a greater degree of soft-tissue support.

Oral hygiene

Problems with oral hygiene are usually recognised by the dentist rather than the patient and often reflect the reasons for tooth loss. High levels of motivation are necessary and the foundations for this must be laid in the treatment planning stages. Poor oral hygiene predisposes to implant failure and some patients need the continued support of a dental hygienist to remove plaque deposits. This can be made more difficult by poor superstructure design and the effective use of hygiene aids must be demonstrated to the patient. Among the devices which are available are interspace brushes, small head tufted brushes, braided floss and non-woven cleaning strips (**6.62–6.69**).

When designing superstructures, it is important to ensure that there are no concavities on the 'fitting' surface which are inaccessible to a brush. Room must also be available to thread the various cleaning aids through the spaces between the implants and between the superstructure and the mucosa.

If professional support in cleaning is required then often this can be achieved without removing the superstructure. A number of aids is now available to assist in cleaning implants, including hard polymeric scalers, which are both effective and cause minimal damage to the surface of the abutment, and specially shaped brushes. If the superstructure has to be removed then, where possible, the gold cylinders should be protected with metal caps whilst cleaning the bridge. Hard deposits can often be readily removed with an acid denture cleaner and any final polishing which might be needed carried out in a dental lathe (**9.36–9.38**).

Refurbishing restorations

The rebasing of implant-stabilised dentures is essentially similar to that of conventional prostheses with special allowance for the retainers.

Where the denture is stabilised by individual attachments, usually of the ball and socket type, the procedure is similar to that for conventional rebasing. After removal of undercuts, the periphery is checked and modified by trimming and border moulding with a suitable viscous material such as greenstick or elastomeric putty. A wash impression is then taken in the denture with a silicone elastomer impression material. This provides enough accuracy for the location of the male attachments. In the laboratory, dummy attachments are placed in the impression and the master cast poured. The denture can then be rebased in the conventional manner and new female attachments located before returning the prosthesis to the clinic. Alternatively, the attachments can be located at the chair side by cutting recesses in the fitting surface of the denture to clear the female components. These are then positioned on the male fixtures together with spacing washers. Finally, self-curing resin is placed in the recesses and the denture fully seated to secure the female attachments in the correct positions. Alternatively, light-curing resin may be used, although this necessitates making a small access hole in the denture on the polished surface. Care must be taken not to overfill the recess with resin and thereby lock the denture to the male attachments.

If an overdenture bar is used then it is preferable if this is picked up in the impression as it provides an accurate record of the relationship of the fixtures in the mouth. If possible, the screws which retain the bar should be replaced with long ones and the denture then perforated over each screw so as to allow it to be seated over the bar. Undercuts are next removed, the periphery of the denture modified as above and the 'tray' loaded with a low viscosity silicone elastomer impression material and fully seated. Once this has set, the screws may be undone and the denture and bar removed. In the laboratory, dummy abutments can be placed on the gold cylinders on the bar and a master cast poured. This then provides all the necessary information for rebasing the denture and relocating the female attachments.

A drawback of the use of long screws is the impossibility of checking the jaw relationship after the impression has been recorded. As a result, it may be prudent to check this before completing the denture. Alternatively, short screws may be used together with a large cap of carding wax over each one to aid its location in the impression. Where the patient is reluctant to be without the denture for several days and a spare is not available then a copy of the current prosthesis may be made in self-curing acrylic resin and used instead.

If an overdenture bar or fixed superstructure framework has fractured then a similar process can be used to obtain a working cast which includes a record of the relationships of the fixtures.

Lost components

Treatment with dental implants involves the intra-oral use of numerous small components, many of which are impossible to secure and difficult to manipulate with gloved hands, whilst protection of the airway with rubber dam is often not practicable. Where design permits, all small tools should be secured to the operator's wrist with a loop of dental floss. Screws may be linked to the end of a screwdriver with carding wax or a length of electrical heat-shrinkable sleeving (**9.39**). As an additional precaution, only the required number of small components should be dispensed and it is preferable if these are placed on the bracket table one at a time so that they may all be accounted for. If a patient is believed to have swallowed or inhaled a component then a careful search must be made of the mouth, protective bib and suction trap in the dental unit. If the object is not found then appropriate radiographs will be required to ensure that it has not been inhaled or lodged in the throat.

Extra-oral fixtures

Difficulties may arise with extra-oral fixtures and these, to a great extent, mirror the problems encountered with intra-oral devices. Failure to integrate, infection and fracture of superstructures may all be encountered. The major problems encountered relate to failure of integration, especially of implants in the orbital rim, soft-tissue problems, orientation difficulties and prosthesis failure. Particular problems arise with fixtures in irradiated bone.

Integration failure

This reflects the difficulty of finding sites with adequate amounts of bone for implant insertion, the relatively small bulk of that bone and the potential for integration to be lost due to mechanical overload and infection. Frequently, the operator's room for manoeuvre is limited by the clinical situation and great care must be taken by both operator and patient to control loading and maintain high levels of hygiene.

Soft-tissue problems

Soft-tissue problems are predominantly related to excessive mobility at the implant site and failure to maintain scrupulous hygiene. Thinning of the soft tissues prior to placing the abutment is often required with ear prostheses.

Orientation difficulties

Whilst the positioning of implants for ear prostheses is relatively straightforward, that for orbital devices is more difficult. Where the fixtures effectively radiate out from the centre of the orbit, access for placing abutments becomes crucial. As a result, recording impressions and placing a superstructure may be very difficult. Careful planning and liaison between surgeon and prosthodontist are essential if difficulties are to be minimised.

Prosthesis failure

Failure of implant-stabilised prostheses is similar to that which occurs with conventional devices and usually results from edge failure or fracture of retainers. Because there is no need to use adhesives, prosthetic materials usually have a greater service life than those used with conventional prostheses.

Surgical problems

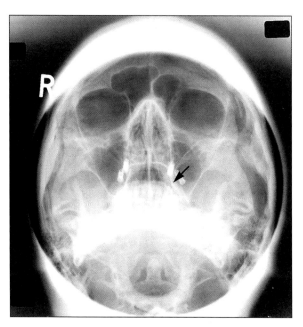

9.1 The implant (arrowed) shown here has become displaced into the maxillary antrum prior to second-stage surgery.

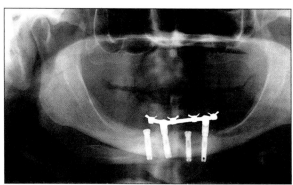

9.2 The fixtures shown here are too long and transfix the mandible.

Infection

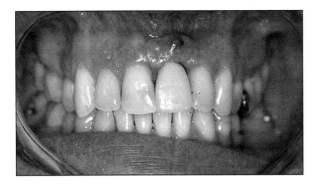

9.3 This patient has an abscess, which has pointed labially, associated with a loose abutment on an implant in the 21 region.

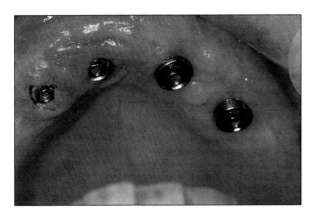

9.4 The tissues around the implants in the 13 and 11 regions are very inflamed as a result of loose abutment screws.

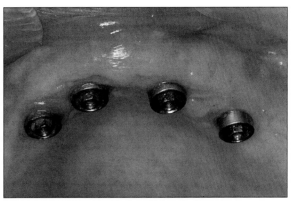

9.5 Clinical picture of the patient shown in 9.4, demonstrating the improvement in tissue health one week after tightening the upper abutment screws.

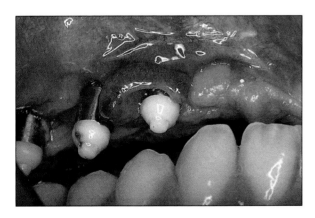

9.6 Inflammation of the soft tissue adjacent to a recently placed abutment. This was associated with a retained suture.

Failure of integration

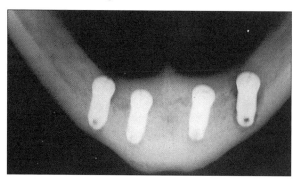

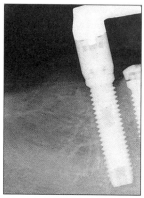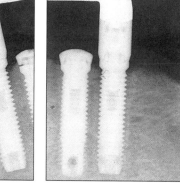

9.7 The implant in the 33 region has failed to integrate. Note the clear radiolucent area around the fixture.

9.8 The radiographic appearances of failure of osseointegration as seen here may be less marked than in 9.6, although there is still an apparent loss of contact between bone and implant.

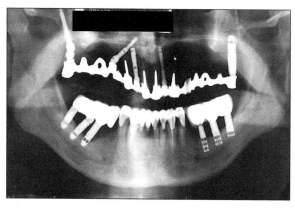

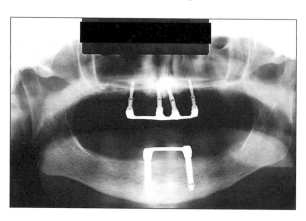

9.9 Failure of osseointegration in the long term is often characterised by loss of crestal bone, which can be severe as seen here, as well as by a radio-lucency around the implant.

9.10 This patient's maxillary implants had suffered severe loss of supporting bone and were very mobile.

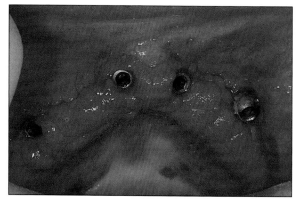

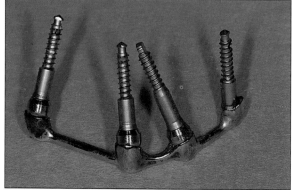

9.11, 9.12 Clinical view of the patient is shown in 9.9. The implants and their associated superstructure were removed as a unit.

Fixture location

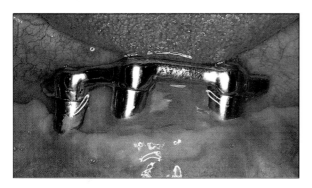

9.13 These implants have been placed too far lingually, causing problems with the soft tissues in the floor of the mouth. The overdenture will need to be set considerably labial to the bar.

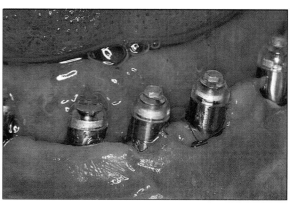

9.14 These implants have not been placed vertically in the bone in the lower jaw and could, with benefit, have been more widely spaced.

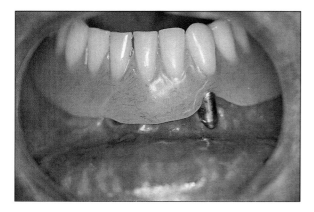

9.15 The implant in the 33 region has been placed too far labially and as a result the denture has had to be reduced in this region so as to prevent excessive bulkiness.

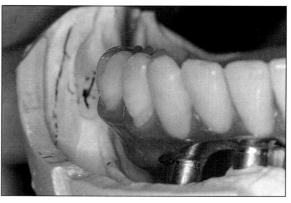

9.16 The need to cantilever markedly the teeth on this prosthesis as a result of misplacement of the implants is evident on the master cast.

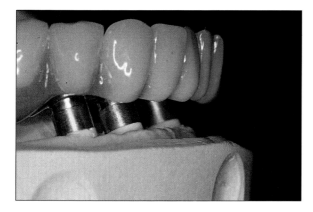

9.17 These implants have been placed too far lingually and retroclined. As a result the lingual aspect of the prosthesis is too bulky and it has had to be markedly cantilevered labially.

Soft-tissue problems

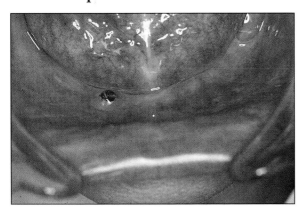

9.18 The soft tissues overlying this fixture have broken down, after first-stage surgery, to expose the cover screw.

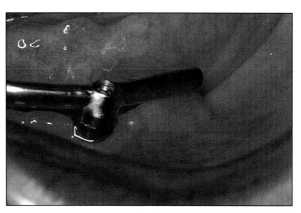

9.19 The soft tissue on the ridge crest has enlarged to obliterate the space below this distally cantilevered bar, which stabilises an overdenture.

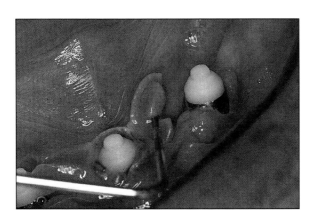

9.20 These implants are used to stabilise a complete overdenture which is retained with a bar and clips. The soft tissues below the bar have enlarged due to mechanical irritation.

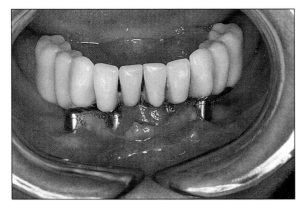

9.21 The soft tissues below this fixed superstructure have enlarged, particularly in the 32 region, due to poor plaque control.

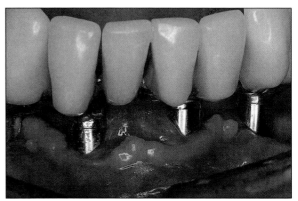

9.22 This close-up view of the implant superstructure shown in 9.19 demonstrates the considerable improvement in tissue contour, which can be produced by improved oral hygiene.

Worn and fractured components

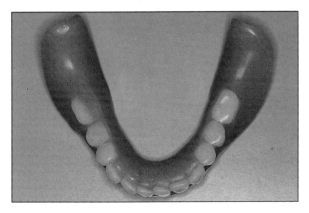

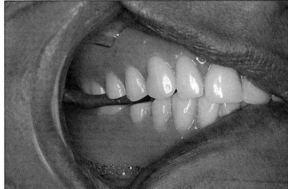

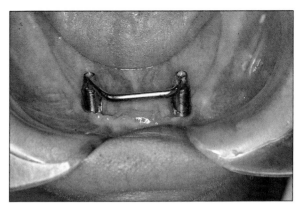

9.23–9.25 This patient uses an implant-stabilised overdenture. As a result of the heavy masticatory loads which she employs, the posterior teeth have been rapidly worn. This has resulted in loss of occlusal contacts. At the same time the occlusal instability has caused tipping of the denture, leading to mucosal trauma and inflammation over the distal denture-bearing areas.

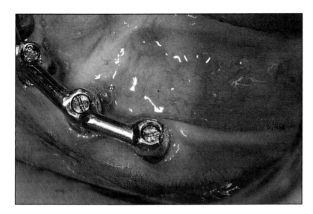

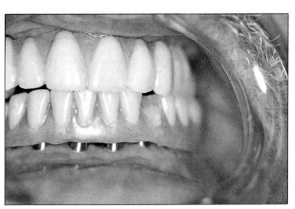

9.26 The distally cantilevered gold bar on this denture-retaining superstructure has fractured through the gold cylinder due to overloading.

9.27 The artificial canine tooth has fractured off this prosthesis due to excessive masticatory loads.

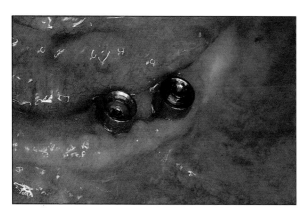

9.28 The head has fractured off the abutment screw on the medial of these two fixtures.

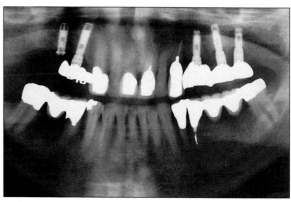

9.29 This radiograph shows an abutment screw which has fractured deep within the fixture. This had probably occurred as a result of excessive masticatory loading in a patient who habitually clenched his teeth.

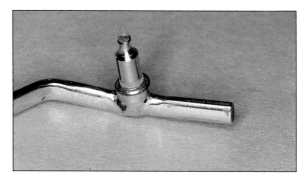

9.30 The abutment screw holding this super-structure fractured close to the top of the fixture and was successfully removed with a probe. This view shows the screw mounted on the gold cylinder with the abutment removed.

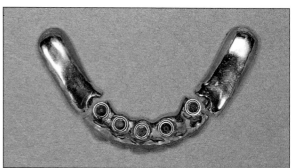

9.31 The cast framework of this fixed superstructure fractured in service due to excessive masticatory loads.

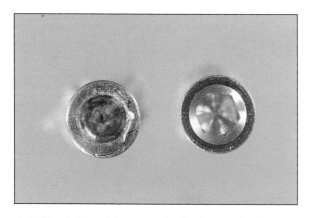

9.32 The internal hexagon in the head of this gold screw has been worn away by injudicious use of a mechanical screwdriver. The wear is evident when the worn screw, on the left, is compared with a new screw.

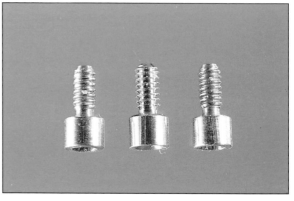

9.33 Repeated tightening and loosening of small screws can result in wear of the threads as seen in the screws on either side of the picture compared with the new one in the centre.

Oral hygiene problems

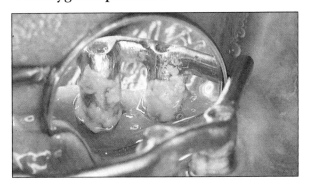

9.34 Poor plaque control on an implant superstructure. Whilst this problem arises more frequently on the lingual aspect of abutments, this patient also had poor plaque control labially.

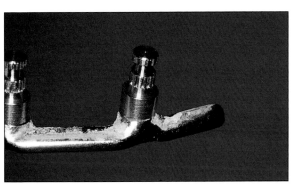

9.35 This patient has found difficulty in keeping the mucosal aspect of this overdenture bar clean, although the other, more accessible, surfaces are plaque-free. Abutment replicas have been placed on the gold cylinders to protect them during cleaning, although their bulk makes them less satisfactory than protective caps (9.37).

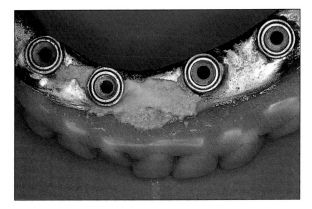

9.36 Heavy calculus deposits on the inferior surface of a fixed superstructure.

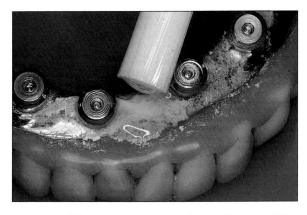

9.37 An acidic denture cleanser is an effective aid in calculus removal. Protective caps have been placed on the gold cylinders and the cleaner is being applied with a brush.

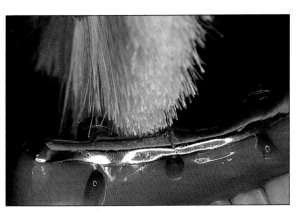

9.38 Final polishing of the superstructure may be conveniently carried out in a lathe.

Lost components

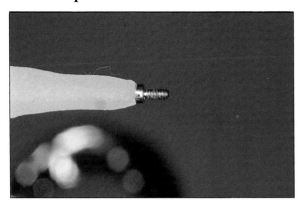

9.39 Carding wax can provide a convenient method of handling small screws.

Extra-oral fixtures

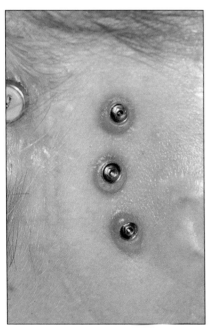

9.40 Chronic inflammation of the soft tissues around osseointegrated implants used to stabilise an artificial ear.

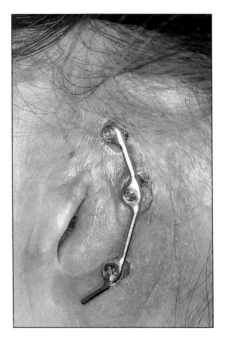

9.41 Occasionally, episodes of acute infection arise in the soft tissues adjacent to extra-oral fixtures.

References

1. Principles of Osseointegration

1. Albrektsson, T. & Albrektsson, B. Osseointegration of bone implants. A review of an alternative mode of fixation. Acta Orthop Scand 58:567–577, 1987
2. Albrektsson, T. & Sennerby, L. State of the art in oral implants. J Clin Periodontol 18:478–481, 1991.
3. Albrektsson, T., Brånemark, P-I., Hansson, H-A. & Lindström, J. Osseointegrated titanium implants. Requirements for ensuring a long-lasting direct bone anchorage in man. Acta Orthop Scand 52:155–170, 1981.
4. Albrektsson, T., Jansson, T. & Lekholm, U. Osseo-integrated dental implants. Dental Clinics of North America 30:151–177, 1986.
5. Albrektsson, T., Johansson, C. & Sennerby, L. Biological aspects of implant dentistry. To be printed in Periodontology 2000 (Lang, N.P., ed.).
6. Brånemark, P-I., Adell, R., Breine, U., Hansson, B-O., Lindström, J. & Ohlsson, Å. Intra-osseous anchorage of dental prostheses I. Experimental studies. Scand J Plast Reconstr Surg 3:81–100, 1969.
7. Frost, H. The biology of fracture healing. An overview for clinicians. Part I and part II. Clin Ort Rel Res 248:283–293 and 294–309. 1989.
8. Hulth, A. Fracture healing. A concept of competing healing factors. Acta Orthop Scand 51:5–7, 1980.
9. Kasemo, B. & Lausmaa, J. Surface science aspects on inorganic biomaterials. CRC Critical Reviews in Biocompatibility 2:335–380, 1986.
10. Mohan, S. & Baylink, D.J. Bone Growth Factors. Clin Orthop Rel Res 263, 30–48, 1991.
11. Wirthlin, R.M. Growth substances: Potential use in periodontics. Journal of Western Society of Periodontology 37:101–125, 1989.
Zarb, G.A. & Albrektsson, T. Osseointegration – A requiem for the periodontal ligament? An editorial. Int & Periodont Restorative Dent 11:88–91, 1991.

2. Anatomical Considerations

Albrektsson, T., Brånemark, P-I., Hansson, H. A., & Lindström, J. Osseointegrated titanium implants. Requirements for ensuring a long-lasting, direct bone-to-implant anchorage in man. Acta. Orthop. Scand. 52:155–70, 1981.
Attwood, D. A. Reduction of residual ridges: a major disease entity. J. Prosth. Dent. 26:266–79, 1971.
Brunski, J. B. Biomechanical Factors Affecting the Bone-Dental Implant Interface. Clinical Materials. 10:153–201, 1992.
Caselman, J. W., Quiryen, M., Lemahieu, S.F., Baert, A. L. & Bonte, J. Computed tomography in the determination of anatomical landmarks in the perspective of endosseous oral implant installation. J. Head Neck Pathology. 7:255–264, 1988.

Hobkirk, J. & Schwab, J. Mandibular deformation in subjects with osseointegrated implants. International Journal of Oral and Maxillofacial Implants. 6:319–328, 1991.
Picton, D. C. A., and Wills, D. J. Viscoelastic properties of the periodontal ligament and mucous membrane. J. Prosthet. Dent. 40:263–272, 1978.
Schwarz, M. S., Rothman, S. L. G., Chafetz, N. & Rhodes, M. Computed tomography in dental implantation surgery. Dent. Clin. N. Amer. 33(4):555–597, 1989.
Tallgren, A. The continuing reduction of the residual alveolar ridges in complete denture wearers: a mixed longitudinal study covering 25 years. J. Prosthet. Dent. 27:120–132, 1972.

3. Selecting an Implant System

Albrektsson, T., Zarb, G.A., Worthington, P., & Eriksson, A.R. The long term efficacy of currently used dental implants: A review and proposed criteria of success. Int. J. Oral and Maxillofac. Implants. 1:11–25, 1986.
Block, M. S., Finger, I., Fontenot, M. G. & Kent, J. N. Loaded hydroxylapatite-coated and grit-blasted titanium implants in dogs. Int. J. Oral and Maxillofac. Implants. 4:219–225, 1989.
Brunski, J. B. Biomaterials and biomechanics in the design of dental implants. Int. J. Oral and Maxillofac. Implants. 3:85–97, 1988.
English, C. E. An overview of implant hardware. J. Am. Dent. Assoc.121:360–368, 1990.
Naert, I., Quiryen, M., van Steenberghe, D., & Darius, P. A comparative study between Brånemark and IMZ implants supporting overdentures: prosthetic considerations. in Tissue integration in Oral, Orthopedic and Maxillo-facial reconstruction. Eds. Laney, W.R. and Tolman, D.E. Quintessence, Chicago. pp 179–193, 1990.

4. Patient Assessment

Cawood, J. & Howell, R. A classification of edentulous jaws. Int. J. Oral and Maxillofac. Surg. 17:232–236, 1988.
Lekholm, U., Zarb, G. A. Patient selection and preparation in Brånemark P.I., Zarb, G. A., Albrektsson, T. (Eds) Tissue Integrated Prostheses: Osseointegration in Clinical Dentistry, Chicago: Quintessence:199–209, 1985.
Sethi, A. Precise site location for implants using CT scans: A technical Note. Int. J. Oral and Maxillofac. Implants. 8:433–438, 1993.
Schwarz, M. S., Rothman, S. L., Rhodes, M. L. & Chafetz, N. Computerised Tomography. Part i: Pre-operative assessment of the mandible for endosseous implant surgery. Part ii: Pre-operative assessment of the maxilla for endosseous implant surgery Int. J. Oral and Maxillofc. Implants. 2:137–141, 2:143–148, 1987.

5. Implant-Stabilised Complete Overdentures

Dahlin, C., Lekholm, U., & Linde, A. A membrane induced bone augmentation at titanium implants. A report of 10 fixtures followed from 1–3 years. Int. J. Periodont. Rest. Dent. 11:273–81, 1991.

Johns, R. B., Jemt, T., Heath, M. R., Watson, R. M. et al. A multicentre study of overdentures supported by Brånemark implants. Int. J. Oral and Maxillofac. Implants. 7:513–522, 1992.

Merickse-Stern, R. & Zarb, G. A. Overdentures: An alternative implant methodology for edentulous patients. Int. J. Prosthodont. 6:203–208, 1993.

Naert, I., Quirynen, M., Theuniers, G. & van Steenberghe, D. Prosthetic aspects of osseointegrated fixtures supporting overdentures. A 4 year report. J. Prosthetic Dent. 65:671–680, 1991.

6. Implant-Stabilised Fixed Prostheses

Adell, R., Lekholm, U., Rockler, B., & Brånemark, P-I. A 15-year study of osseointegrated implants in the treatment of the edentulous jaw. Int. J. Oral Surg. 10:387–416, 1981.

Albrektsson, T., Dahl, E., Enbom, L., Engevall, S., Enquist B., Ericsson A.R., et al. Osseointegrated oral implants. A Swedish multicenter study of 8139 consecutively inserted Nobelpharma implants. J. Periodontol 59:287–296, 1988.

Blomberg S., Brånemark P-I. & Carlsson G.E. Psychological reactions to edentulousness and treatment with jawbone anchored bridges. Acta. Psychiatr. Scand. 68:251–262, 1984.

Davis, D.M. The role of implants in the treatment of edentulous patients. Int. J. Prosthodont. 3:42–50, 1990.

Hobkirk, J.A. & Psarros, K. The influence of Occlusal Surface Material on Peak Masticatory forces Using Osseointegrated Implant-Supported Prostheses. Int. J. Oral and Maxillofacial Implants. 7:345-352, 1992.

van Steenberghe D. The impact of osseointegrated prostheses on treatment planning in oral rehabilitation. In: Albrektsson T., Zarb G.A., (Eds) The Brånemark Osseointegrated Implant. Chicago: Qintessence, 139-145, 1989.

7. The Partially Edentulous Patient

Ekfeldt, A., Carlsson, G. and Borjesson, G. Clinical evaluation of single tooth restorations supported by osseointegrated implants: A retrospective study. Int. J. Oral and Maxillofac. Implants. 9:179–183, 1994,

Ericsson I., Lekholm U., Brånemark P-I., Lindhe, J., Glantz, P-O. & Nyman, S. A clinical evaluation of fixed bridge restorations supported by the combination of teeth andosseointegrated titanium implants. J. Clin. Periodontol. 13:307–312, 1986.

Ericsson I., Glantz P.O., & Brånemark P-I. Use of implants in restorative dentistry in patients with reduced periodontal tissue support. Qintessence Int. 19:801–807, 1988.

Israelson, H. & Plemons, J.M. Dental implants, regenerative techniques and periodontal plastic surgery. Int. J. Oral and Maxillofac. Implants. 8:555–561, 1993.

Jemt, T. & Lekholm, U. Oral implant treatment in posterior partially edentulous jaws: A 5 year follow-up report. Int. J. Oral and Maxillofac. Implants. 8:635–640, 1993.

Laney, W. R., Jemt, T., Harris, D., Henry, P. J., Krogh, P. H., Polizzi, G., Zarb, G. & Hermann, I. Osseointegrated implants for single tooth replacement: Progress report from a multicentre prospective study after 3 years. Int. J. Oral and Maxillofac. Implants. 9:49–54, 1994.

Parel, S.M. & Sullivan, D.Y. (Eds). Esthetics and Osseointegration. Taylor Publishing Company, Dallas. Osseointegration Seminars Inc., 1989.

Zarb, G. A., Zarb, F.L., & Schmitt, A. Osseointegrated implants for partially edentulous patients. Dent. Clin. North Amer. 31(3):457–472, 1987.

8. Maxillo-Facial Implants

Henry, P. Maxillofacial prosthetic considerations in advanced osseointegration surgery. Worthington, P. & Brånemark, P-I., (Eds). Illinois: Quintessence Publishing Company. 24:313–326.

Parel, S.M. & Tjellström, A. The United States and Swedish experience with osseointegrated and facial prostheses. Int. J. Oral and Maxillofac. Implants. 6:75–79, 1991.

Thomas, K. Prosthetic rehabilitation. Quintessence Publishing Company Ltd, London., 1994.

Tjellstrom, A., Jansson, K., & Brånemark, P-I. Craniofacial defects in advanced osseointegration surgery. Worthington, P. and Brånemark, P-I. (Eds).Quintessence Publishing Company, Illinois. 25:293–312, 1992.

Tjellström, A., Yontchev, S., Lindström, J. et al. Five years experience with bone-anchored auricular prostheses. Otolaryngol. Head Neck Surg. 93(3):366–372, 1985.

Watson, R. M., Coward, T. J., Forman, G. H. & Moss, J. P. Considerations in treatment planning for implant supported auricular prostheses. Int. J. Oral and Maxillofac. Implants. 8:688–694, 1993.

9. Problems

Hemmings, K. W., Schmitt, A. & Zarb, G. A. Complications and maintenance requirements for fixed prostheses and overdentures in the edentulous mandible: A 5 Year Report. Int. J. Oral and Maxillofac. Implants. 9:191–196, 1994.

Jemt, T. Failures and complications in 391 consecutively inserted fixed prostheses supported by Brånemark implants in edentulous jaws: A study from the time of prosthesis placement to the first annual check-up. Int. J. Oral and Maxillofac. Implants. 6:270–275, 1991.

Worthington, P., Bolender, C. and Taylor, T. The Swedish system of osseointegrated implants: Problems and complications encountered in a four year trial period. Int. J. Oral and Maxillofac. Implants. 2:77–84, 1987.

Zarb, G.A. & Schmitt, A. The longitudinal clinical effectiveness of osseointegrated dental implants. The Toronto Study Part III. Problems and complications encountered. J. Prosthet. Dent. 64:185–194, 1990.

Index